NONE
OF THESE
DISEASES

NONE
OF THESE
DISEASES

THE BIBLE'S HEALTH SECRETS
FOR THE 21ST CENTURY

S. I. McMillen, M.D.
and David E. Stern, M.D.

―――――――――Millennium Three Edition―――――――――

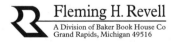

Fleming H. Revell
A Division of Baker Book House Co
Grand Rapids, Michigan 49516

Published by Revell
a division of Baker Publishing Group
P.O. Box 6287, Grand Rapids, MI 49516-6287
www.revellbooks.com

Printed in the United States of America

Library of Congress Cataloging-in-Publication Data
McMillen, S. I. (Sim I.) 1898–
    None of these diseases : the Bible's health secrets for the 21st century /
S. I. McMillen & David E. Stern.—3rd ed.
      p.   cm.
    "Millennium three edition."
    Includes bibliographical references.
    ISBN 10: 0-8007-5719-X
    ISBN 978-0-8007-5719-9
    1. Health—Biblical teaching. 2. Medicine—Biblical teaching.
3. Health—Religious aspects—Christianity. 4. Medicine—Religious
aspects—Christianity. I. Title.
BS680.H413 M37 2000
613—dc21   99-059836

14   15   14   13   12   11

Contents

Part 5 Spiritual Wholeness

PART 1

THE SOURCE
OF WHOLENESS

ONE

Eel Eyes and Goose Guts

Rx: _____

Name: _____

Date: *1500 B.C.* _____

To cure pinkeye apply the urine of a faithful wife.

Dr. _____

This prescription comes from the famous *Ebers Papyrus,* a medical book from 1500 B.C. Of course this treatment was useless and dangerous. But if the pinkeye did not get better fast, the poor woman probably had to explain herself.

The *Ebers Papyrus* gives us a picture of medicine in ancient Egypt, that day's most advanced civilization. To cure baldness, doctors applied "a mixture of six fats . . . [from] the horse, the hippopotamus, the crocodile, the cat, the snake, and the [wild goat]."[1] All that grease grew few hairs, but at least it shined the hairless dome.

The *Ebers Papyrus* lists hundreds of prescriptions, with an amazing array of ingredients: statue dust, beetle shells, mouse tails, cat hair, pig eyes, dog toes, breast milk, human semen, eel eyes, and goose guts. The best one can say about these medications is that at least they were "100 percent natural."

Good and Laudable Pus

To splinters, the ancient Egyptian doctors applied a salve of worm blood and donkey dung. Since dung is loaded with tetanus spores, a simple splinter often resulted in a gruesome death from lockjaw.

Until the late 1800s, however, most doctors thought pus promoted healing. Thus doctors infected wounds to get them to produce pus. They agreed with the Ebers Papyrus: "It is good for a wound to rot a little. . . . Therefore, put something in the wound that will [make it produce pus]."[2]

A modern doctor comments on the *Ebers Papyrus:*

[This is] the first known statement of the dirtiest, messiest, most pernicious, and most persistent mistake in the history of surgery: getting the badness out of a wound. . . . It has been among the catchiest concepts in the history of medicine. . . . Rivers of pus flowed for another 3,500 years, and the dreadful doctrine of good and laudable pus . . . has only recently faded.[3]

In the ancient world, well-meaning doctors killed millions by deliberately infecting their wounds.

Moses and Medicine

Moses lived in Egypt while the Egyptian doctors were writing this medical text. Raised in the royal court, he "was educated in all the wisdom of the Egyptians" (Acts 7:22). No doubt, he knew and used the Egyptian remedies.

Moses had been steeped in these infection-spreading practices. Who would expect Moses to make breakthroughs in epidemic prevention? Yet Moses recorded an unlikely promise to the ancient Hebrews:

> If you give careful attention to the voice of the Lord your God, do what is right in his sight, give ear to his commandments, and keep all his statutes, I will put none of these diseases upon you, which I have brought upon the Egyptians; for I am the Lord who heals you.
>
> Exodus 15:26

"None of these diseases!" What a promise! For centuries epidemics had killed thousands of Egyptians and Hebrews. Ancient treatments rarely helped. Often the "cure" was worse than the disease. Yet here God made a fantastic promise—freedom from diseases.

God then gave Moses many health rules, filling a whole section of the Bible. Would Moses have enough faith to record the divine innovations, even if they contradicted his royal postgraduate university training? If Moses had yielded to his natural tendency to add even a little of his "higher education," the Bible would contain such prescriptions as "urine of a faithful wife" or "blood of a worm." We might even expect him to prescribe the "latest" animal manure concoction. But the record is clear. Moses recorded hundreds of health regulations but not a single current medical misconception.

Thousands have died through the centuries, however, because doctors ignored the biblical rules. Finally, when doctors read and tried these guidelines, they quickly discovered how to prevent the spread of epidemics. Thus Moses could be called the father of modern infection control.

Even today we are still benefiting from God's 3,500-year-old instructions.

TWO

Back to the Breakthrough

Following the precepts laid down in Leviticus, the church . . . accomplished the first great feat . . . in methodical eradication of disease.

George S. Rosen, M.D.

From across the room, I (SIM) knew his terrible diagnosis. Five years earlier the disease had started as a white patch on his arm. Over the years it had deformed and paralyzed his hands. His fingers and toes had rotted away, leaving ulcer-covered stumps. The disease had left him blind.

His parents, having carried him through the jungles for three days to see me, now desperately looked to me for a cure. But it was 1932. He had leprosy. Medical science had little to offer.

Such intense suffering placed a heavy load on my heart. What I had, I gave—a cleansing of his wounds and a prayer for God's touch. To keep the leprosy from spreading to the rest of his family, I applied a prescription written by Moses over 3,500 years earlier.

The AIDS of the Dark Ages

For centuries leprosy killed millions. Dr. George Rosen describes the horror of leprosy's slow, mutilating death:

> Leprosy cast the greatest blight that threw its shadow over the daily life of medieval humanity. Fear of all other diseases taken together can hardly be compared to the terror spread by leprosy. Not even the Black Death . . . or the appearance of syphilis . . . produced a similar state of fright.[1]

What did doctors think caused leprosy? Some taught that it was brought on by eating spicy food, spoiled fish, or diseased pork. Others said it was caused by "malign conjunctions of the planets." Naturally their ideas for preventing the spread of leprosy never worked.

How did Europe try to bring the leprosy epidemic under control? Dr. Rosen gives us the answer: "Leadership was taken by the church, as the physicians had nothing to offer."[2]

Could the church of the Dark Ages succeed where doctors had failed? Could so-called backward ministers lead medical science forward? In fact ministers looked back—back almost 3,500 years to the writings of Moses.

Saved from Every Sickness

Remember, Moses was fully educated in ancient Egyptian superstitions. Ancient Egyptians thought epidemics were caused by "disease demons," so they cast spells to protect themselves.

One formula is written in the *Smith Papyrus*, dating from around the time of Moses. It was for protection against epidemics. It was to be chanted while a person had two vulture feathers held over him:

O Flame-in-His-Face! . . . O Nekhbet, lifting the earth to the sky
for her father, come thou, bind the two feathers around me, around
me, that I may live and flourish because I possess this White One.
. . . O Seizer-of-the-Great-One, son of Sekhmet, mightiest of the
mighty, son of the Disease-Demon, . . . flooder of the streams; when
thou voyagest in the Celestial Ocean, when thou sailest in the
morning barque, thou hast saved me from every sickness.[3]

What a promise! *"Saved . . . from every sickness."* When Moses
attended the University of Egypt, his professor also promised
"none of these diseases." But Egypt's mummies are riddled with
diseases, so we can be sure that this formula did not "save . . .
from every sickness."

The editor of the *Smith Papyrus* excuses these superstitious
doctors by noting that they were "inevitably . . . children of their
time."[4]

Was Moses "inevitably a child of his time"? Did he provide
the Hebrews with a spell to stop epidemics? Read his ancient
prescription: "As long as he has leprosy . . . he must live alone
outside the camp" (Lev. 13:46). There was not even a trace of
superstition. This ancient order clearly states the modern concept of quarantine.

One historian notes, "The laws against leprosy in Leviticus
13 may be regarded as the first model of a sanitary legislation."[5]
Indeed, the biblical method makes a radical break from all
ancient concepts of disease. No superstition. No leprosy
demons. No animal dung salve.

Maybe we should seriously consider Moses' claim to have
received these teachings directly from God.

Norway's Desperate Experiment

In the ignorance of the late 1700s, a leprosy epidemic raged
in Norway. The people were so desperate that they finally listened to their preachers and carefully followed the biblical
rules. By the early 1800s, Norway's leprosy epidemic was under
control. But they were not completely sure why the epidemic

had faded. Maybe the epidemic was just running its natural course. Maybe the biblical precautions had no real effect.

Most Norwegians thought that leprosy was hereditary. They did not know it could spread from person to person. Thus they had no fear of contact with lepers.

As the fear of epidemic faded, Norway relaxed the precautions. Lepers were no longer isolated. Lepers even specialized in door-to-door sales—spreading disease from house to house.[6]

Once again the epidemic flared out of control.

The 3,500-Year-Old Secret

In 1873, however, Dr. Armauer Hansen looked through a microscope at a slide from a leprosy patient. The tiny red dots he saw thrust the world out of the Dark Ages of leprosy. The tiny red dots were the leprosy bacteria. Finally, people realized that leprosy was an infection. It was passed from person to person.

Millions of leprosy bacteria live in the nose.[7] You can catch leprosy from a simple sneeze in the face. Leprosy bacteria can even live dried out for several days.[8] Thus you can even catch leprosy from eating off an unwashed plate.

After 3,500 years, science had discovered the secret of quarantine. Separating infected patients would stop the spread of leprosy. Norway enacted the Norwegian Leprosy Act, requiring strict enforcement of the biblical precautions. In less than sixty years, Norway's leper count dropped from 2,858 to 69. Eventually the great discoveries of science allowed Norway to wipe out leprosy.

Many countries began to practice God's command. "As long as he has the infection . . . he must live alone outside the camp" (Lev. 13:46). Soon much of the world was free of leprosy—a disease that had ravaged humanity for centuries. Dr. Rosen notes:

> The church took as its guiding principle the concept of contagion as embodied in the Old Testament. . . . This idea and its practical consequences are defined with great clarity in the book of Leviticus. . . . Once the priest had diagnosed leprosy, the indi-

vidual had to live in protective quarantine, segregated from the community.

Following the precepts laid down in Leviticus the church undertook the task of combating leprosy; . . . [and] it accomplished the first great feat . . . in methodical eradication of disease.[9]

They experienced the promise of God: "If you will give careful attention to the voice of the Lord your God . . . I will put none of these diseases upon you. . . ."

THREE

A Labor of Love

> I am in the right and so I shall remain as long as the human female continues to bear children.
>
> Ignaz Semmelweis

Imagine you have a time machine and you can travel to anywhere and any time. One day you set the time for May 1847 and the destination for Vienna, Austria. Capital of the Hapsburg Empire, Vienna has been home to Mozart, Mahler, Beethoven, and Brahms. Vienna is a thoroughly modern nineteenth-century city, the world's leading medical center.

When you arrive at the Vienna General Hospital, the morning mist is lifting from the immense court-yard. Walks crisscross azalea-filled flower beds. A young man, wearing a black suit and top hat, heads for the entrance of the hospital. Mumbling as he walks, he is obviously upset.

You follow him through the front door of the hospital building. You wince; the ward smells like a dead animal. Nurses bustle through the corridors. Muffled moans, coughs, and sobs are punctuated by a rare shriek of pain.

You turn the corner and you have entered the morgue. On the other side of the autopsy table, five medical students stand with their sleeves rolled up. On the table is the dead body of a young woman. Your preoccupied friend is the obstetrician Dr. Ignaz Semmelweis. He hangs up his coat and top hat, rolls up his sleeves, and asks, "How many women died last night?" One student speaks, "Three, Josephine Frankle, Marie . . ." You notice a tear in his eye as the intern recites the names.

Dr. Semmelweis shakes his head, "Admission, delivery, death. Is that our motto? One out of six women lying in our delivery beds ends up lying on this autopsy table. I cannot accept this. The women die and we have no idea why. Why? Why?"

The students are casting nervous glances at each other. They obviously have no idea why so many women are dying.

They move to the business at hand. With bare hands the students perform the autopsies one after the other without even a break to wash their hands. The corpses have one thing in common—pus: pus-filled abdomens, pus-filled chests, even a pus-filled eye socket. The diagnosis is the same for each: "labor fever . . . labor fever . . . labor fever."[1]

After the autopsies, the students merely rinse their bloody hands in water, wipe them dry on a rag, and walk off to the maternity ward for morning rounds. Their hands and clothes still stink of rotting flesh.

In the ward many women are simply waiting to go into labor; several are crying from labor pains; one is shivering from a raging fever; one is gasping her last few breaths; one has the ominous sheet pulled over her head.

The students go from bed to bed, asking questions and performing internal exams. Dr. Semmelweis double-checks their findings and makes several teaching points.

Suddenly, you realize a rank reality. Their hands have been in pus, blood, and dead bodies. They have been in pregnant woman after pregnant woman. But no one has yet washed his hands. What are they thinking?

This is the standard practice throughout Europe. No one has even thought of the existence of bacteria, much less seen them. Scientists usually blame epidemics on vague "atmospheric conditions" or "cosmic-telluric influences."

In a moment, that is about to change.

Suddenly, Semmelweis stops rounds. He orders the interns to wash their hands. The interns laugh nervously, thinking at first it's a joke. But Dr. S. is not much of a joker. He is serious— intensely serious.

Someone finds a basin, and Semmelweis watches each one wash in heavily chlorinated water. He sniffs their hands to make sure the smell is gone. Then he announces his theory. He suspects the cause of labor fever may be on their hands. Maybe their hands are carrying labor fever from the dead to the living. The so-called modern medical care may actually be killing the women. To you this seems painfully obvious; you don't need "M.D." after your name to know you should wash your hands after doing an autopsy. But remember, no one suspects that diseases can be transmitted from one person to another.[2]

Semmelweis then tells the students the evidence for his theory:

- Women who have more internal exams are more likely to die of labor fever.
- Recently his friend Dr. Jakob Kolletschka had suddenly died of blood poisoning from an inflamed finger cut—a cut he had suffered while performing an autopsy of a woman killed by labor fever. At his autopsy they found pus in the abdomen, pus in the chest, pus on the brain, and pus-pockets in the skin. If he had been a new mother, his diagnosis would have been labor fever. He must have caught it from the woman's corpse.
- If a doctor delivers the baby, the death rate is 18 percent. If a midwife attends the labor, the death rate is only 3 percent. Physicians do autopsies; midwives do not. Maybe the

difference is in the autopsies. Maybe doctors are carrying a lethal substance from dead bodies to living women.

Everything seems to point to the same conclusion. The filth on the doctors' hands is killing the women.

One skeptical student reminds him of his last theory. While ringing a bell, the priest had been entering the ward to administer last rites at all hours of the night. Semmelweis had suspected that this morbid commotion was literally scaring the women to death. Thus he made the priest enter silently through a side door. But the death rate remained sky high. Why should washing their hands be any different?

Another student remembers Semmelweis's idea that turning the women onto their sides might lower the death rate. They performed deliveries with the women lying on their sides, but it had no effect on labor fever.

"We know what doesn't work," Semmelweis says. "We must find what will work. Let's wash and wait. We shall see what happens."

Wash and Wait

The history books tell us what happened next. Labor fever virtually disappeared from the ward. In just three months, the death rate fell from 18 percent to 1 percent.

His findings were published in a medical journal, but hardly anyone noticed. Everyone laughed at the doctor who thought hand washing might be as important as laxatives and ventilating rooms.

Back to the Scripture

Semmelweis had made one of the most important discoveries in the history of medicine—isolating dead bodies from healthy people. But this idea did not originate with Semmelweis. Three thousand years earlier, God said to Moses, "Whoever touches any dead body will be off-limits[3] for seven days" (Num. 19:11). Those declared "off-limits" had to take a shower of cleansing before they could reenter the community.

"Off-limits," what did that mean? It meant that if you touched a dead body, you would have to leave your home, leave your job, and spend an entire week alone in the surrounding desert (Num. 5:2–3). The ancient Hebrews avoided becoming off-limits at all costs. They did not touch the dead body, and the disease-causing bacteria died with the corpse.

What a contrast from the customs of Egypt, where Moses had spent the first forty years of his life! Egyptians made mummies of dead bodies. Here is a textbook description of the procedure. Remember, they did all this with their bare hands.

> The process of mummification consisted of extracting the brain through the nose; removing the lungs and the abdominal organs . . . through an incision cut in the left flank; placing the body in [a preservative]; and finally wrapping the body in many layers of bandages. . . . The internal organs were sometimes embalmed separately and put in four . . . jars.[4]

During the embalming process, many people put their hands in the dead body. The germs that killed the corpse covered their hands. Then they went out and spread the germs to the market, to their friends, and even to their families. No wonder the Egyptians were a people of epidemics.

Once again, Moses completely ignored his Egyptian upbringing. By prohibiting touching of the dead, he ended the process of embalming. Instead of spreading germs to the living, the dead body took its germs six feet under.

Semmelweis was right; hand washing after touching the dead saved lives. The Bible had gone one better. Never touching the dead would save more lives.

Just how advanced were the biblical rules? Even during the early 1980s at the Philadelphia City Morgue, many workers refused to wear gloves and still did autopsies with their bare hands. When my (DES) wife questioned them about this, they seemed completely unafraid of catching disease.

The Disgrace of Discovery

Let's go back to Dr. Semmelweis. One day the doctors and students examined a row of twelve women. Eleven of the twelve caught labor fever and died. Semmelweis's alert brain gave birth to another new idea; maybe doctors' hands could transfer labor fever from one living woman to another living woman. He ordered a new routine. Doctors must wash their hands after every internal examination—no exceptions.

If he seemed silly before, now he became the crazy Dr. Clean Freak. Students howled in protest. "Washing, washing, washing . . . What a nuisance . . . My hands are chapped . . . They stink of chlorine . . ."

Despite their protests, the death rate dropped even further.

Even the father of cellular pathology, Dr. Rudolf Virchow, ridiculed Semmelweis. The faculty clung to their own false theories of labor fever's causes: constipation, late lactation, panic attacks, or bad air.

His colleagues challenged, "How can something as simple as washing hands prevent something as severe as labor fever?" When he tried to defend hand washing, they simply laughed him off.

His boss staunchly held to the bad air theory, so he felt that Semmelweis was being disrespectful. He bad-mouthed Semmelweis to the students and faculty. He had Semmelweis demoted. Finally, he fired him.

His successor threw out the washbasins; up shot the death rate. Again the cries of dying women filled the maternity ward. Were his colleagues convinced then? Not at all! The power of pride and prejudice blinded them to the proof.

For eight months Dr. Semmelweis struggled to find another job. But Dr. Clean Freak had been blackballed. Finally, the hospital offered him a teaching position but prohibited him from seeing patients. Semmelweis's greatest joy was delivering healthy babies. He was a doctor. He had to practice medicine.

Shocked and depressed, he left Vienna without saying good-bye to his few friends.

Traveling 135 miles down the Danube River, he went home to Budapest. He found a job in a local hospital, where the cries of dying women echoed in the maternity ward. Semmelweis brought back the washbasins. Again the grim reaper's harvest ended. Semmelweis was ecstatic. He had duplicated his results. He had proven his theory. Now they would have to listen. But once again, pride and prejudice blinded his colleagues. Some even passed him in the halls without speaking.

He outlined his findings in a 543-page book, but most of his jealous peers did not even read it. Thousands of lives could have been saved, but the establishment would not listen. The more he shared his theory, the more they ridiculed it.

Dr. Carl Braun, who had once practiced with Semmelweis, denounced the theory in his famous *Textbook of Obstetrics:* "In Germany, France and England, this hypothesis of cadaveric infection has been condemned almost unanimously up to this day."[5]

Frustrated and furious, Semmelweis could no longer hold in his anger. Truth was not a democracy. The majority could just as easily agree on error as truth, especially if they refused to look at the truth. Semmelweis publicly denounced a doctor who disagreed with him: "Your teaching . . . is based upon the dead bodies of new mothers slaughtered through ignorance. I denounce you before God and the world as a murderer, and the History of Labor Fever will . . . perpetuate your name as a medical Nero."

The death cries of new mothers so haunted and weighed on the sensitive nature of Dr. Semmelweis that his sanity finally broke. His family committed him to a mental institution. There at the age of forty-seven, he himself caught blood poisoning and died, ironically, of the very disease he had labored so hard to prevent.

His life's labor of love could have saved millions. His discovery should have made him famous. Instead, he died insane, unknown, and unappreciated. He knew that someday science would recognize and use his great discovery. He wrote, "The conviction that this time will come without fail, sooner or later after me, will still soothe my hour of death."[6]

A Time to Bond

Centuries before Dr. Semmelweis, God declared any new mother to be off-limits for an entire week (Leviticus 12). No one was allowed to touch her. Anyone who mistakenly touched her was to bathe, wash his clothes, and remain separate until sundown. This strict isolation protected new mothers from catching labor fever.

Some feminists have suggested that this isolation of new mothers reflected a low view of women in a male-dominated society. Maybe it had nothing to do with a low view of women. Maybe it came from God's high view of mothers and motherhood.

Without interruptions, a new mother was left alone to devote that first week to her newborn baby. Psychologists are just beginning to understand the important bonding of mother and baby. Both baby and mother need a strong emotional bond to each other, and the baby's first few days are critical in developing this bonding. Many doctors today recommend a similar rest period for a new mother to bond with her baby.

Wash or Beware

Of course Semmelweis was right about hand washing. Dead people have germs, germs cause disease, and germs spread on hands. Wash the hands and you wash away the germs.

Germs are everywhere. The same bacteria living at the bottom of a cesspool live on windowsills, chairs, and even in the air. Of course in small numbers they are no big deal; but in warm, moist areas, such as our hands, bacteria multiply by the millions.

Even in modern American hospitals, over two million patients catch infections during hospitalization. The vast majority are transmitted on the hands of medical personnel who neglect careful hand washing. What a tragedy—a preventable tragedy! Listen to a modern medical textbook: "Routine hand washing is to be done before, between and after contact with patients. This is the most important feature of infection control." Nothing has changed since the days of Semmelweis.

Semmelweis's method prevented many deaths, but no modern hospital would allow washing in a common bowl of standing water. The Centers for Disease Control (CDC) has outlined the proper method for hand washing. "The hands should be vigorously lathered and rubbed together for 15 seconds, under a moderate-sized stream of water. . . . There is no good substitute for routine hand washing with soap and running water."[7] Let's compare modern hand washing with the biblical method in Numbers 19:

- **Running water:** to rinse off germs.
  Biblical Method: Water was showered from a hyssop branch.
- **Time:** to assure a thorough job.
  Biblical Method: The washings were repeated over a period of seven days. Between washings germs were killed by the sun and by drying.
- **Antiseptic soap:** to kill germs.
  Biblical Method: Hyssop contains the antiseptic thymol,[8] the active ingredient in Listerine.
- **Vigorous scrubbing:** to dislodge germs from crevasses.
  Biblical Method: The soap contained cedar oil, a skin irritant to encourage scrubbing. The soap also contained wool fibers, making it the ancient equivalent of Lava soap. Once the soap was on you, you had to scrub to get it off.

Centuries before Semmelweis, God had already detailed the most effective method of washing. To prevent the spread of disease, modern science has merely rediscovered the biblical method.

Surgery—a Death Sentence

We can only wish that humanity had discovered hand washing sooner. During most of the nineteenth century, patients and doctors prepared for surgery very casually. The patient walked in, undressed, and lay down on the operating table. The surgeon took off his coat, rolled up his sleeves, picked up his black bag, pulled out some instruments, and started to operate. If the surgeon wished his students to examine something, they would simply step forward and poke their germ-covered hands into the gaping wound.

Major surgery usually meant death. The great surgeon Dr. Roswell Park related his experiences:

> When I began my work, in 1876 [twenty-nine years after Semmelweis's discoveries], as a hospital interne, in one of the largest hospitals in this country, . . . during my first winter's experience, with but one or two exceptions, every patient operated upon . . . died of blood poisoning.[9]

Surgeons could have prevented many of these deaths simply by washing their hands. In fact during World War II some hospitals ran out of rubber gloves, so surgeons carefully washed their hands and operated with bare hands. The doctors were astounded when they found that the infection rates did not go up.

Lather and Live

Today no doctor should examine a patient without first scrubbing his or her hands with antiseptic soap. Even so, failure to wash hands carefully still results in many infections.

A few years ago the nursery at Boston City Hospital suffered an outbreak of a bacterial infection. During this outbreak, eleven newborn infants caught the infection and four died. Doctors searched for the source and soon found it—the unwashed hands of a single nurse.[10]

Even today doctors keep rediscovering—at frightful cost—the necessity of antiseptic washing: a principle that God gave to Moses 3,500 years ago.

Semmelweis himself probably would not have been surprised that the Bible had predated his discoveries, for he once wrote, "From all that lives . . . emanates the omnipotence of the divine."

FOUR

To Sewer or Not to Sewer

The Invisible Invasion

In 1847, while Semmelweis was making his great discovery, a savage army threatened England. Starting in Afghanistan, it had already sailed down the rivers of Europe and killed thousands in every city.

The army's troops were trillions of cholera bacteria. They attacked a person explosively. Within hours they could purge a gallon of "rice water" diarrhea—rapidly dehydrating a victim to the edge of death. Patients presented dramatically—blue, pulseless, and writhing from muscle cramps. Over half of these would die.

The epidemic raged on the Continent. England waited in terror.

The Sanitary Man

Parliament turned to Edwin Chadwick, the one man who might defend them against the invisible invasion. On the Board of Health, Chadwick had spent the last fourteen years studying the sicknesses of England.

His findings had startled the nation. He had found that a rich gentleman could expect to live forty-three years, but a poor Englishman averaged only twenty-two years. Why such a wide difference? Chadwick declared that the poor were dying from a lack of sanitation.

During a single year, one medical officer had noticed sixty-three epidemic victims in one courtyard of twelve houses. He reported:

> I found the whole court inundated with fluid filth . . . [oozing] from two adjoining . . . cesspools, which had no means of escape . . . [since they were] below the level of the street, and having no drain. . . . The fever was constantly recurring there. The house nearest the [cesspool] had been [unoccupied] for nearly three years in consequence of the filthy matter oozing up through the floor, and the occupiers of the adjoining houses were unable to take their meals without previously closing the doors and windows.[1]

Underneath the streets ran massive sewer tunnels. Water might trickle across their flat bottoms but it rarely washed them clear. In reality, sewers were nothing more than underground dung heaps.

Every five to ten years, workers dug up the streets and opened the sewers. They climbed down and lifted buckets of solid sewage up to the street. Wagons carted the waste to farms for fertilizer. Then the crops, tainted with human waste, were brought back into the city to be eaten. It would be difficult to design a better system for spreading disease.

With fifty-four signatures, the following letter voiced the plight of thousands:

The Editur of the [London] Times Paper.
Sir,
  May we beg and beseach your proteckshion and power. . . . We live in muck and filthe. We aint got no priviz [outhouses], no dust bins [garbage cans], no drains, no [running] water . . . and no suer in the whole place. The Suer Company . . . all great, rich and powerfool men take no notice watsomedever of our cumplaints. The Stenche of a Gully-hole is disgustin. We al of us suffur, and numbers are ill, and if the Colera comes Lord help us.
  Some gentlemans comed yesterday, and we thought they was comishoners from the suer Company, but they was complaining of the noosance and stenche. . . . They was much surprized to see the seller [cellar] in Number 12 . . . where a child was dyin from fever, and would not beleave that Sixty persons sleep in it every night. This here seller you couldent swing a cat in.
  Praeye Sir com and see us, for we are livin like piggs, and it aint faire we shoulde be so ill treted. . . .[2]

The rich were appalled to hear of such squalor—squalor they never saw because they stayed out of these neighborhoods. They lived in homes with running water, toilets, and garbage service. Chadwick's newspaper articles forced them to face the misery of the other side of London.

Still, the rich insisted that the sicknesses of poverty resulted from "voluntary" laziness: neglecting hygiene, drinking alcohol, avoiding doctors, and crowding together.

Chadwick disagreed. What was "voluntary" about living, working, and sleeping in your own sewage? The sewage kept them constantly sick. Constantly sick, they died young. Dying young, they left orphans. The cycle of poverty, sewage, sickness, and death continued from generation to generation.

Chadwick had found the problem and he had also devised a solution. He had shown that every house could receive running water, a flush toilet, a draining sewer, and garbage collection— all for less than a penny a day. He ridiculed the notion that the best one could do was charity—handing out a few sandwiches, blankets, and pennies. Money was wasted on this so-called charity. What good were sandwiches to sixty people stuffed into a filthy windowless basement and wallowing in human waste? They needed sewers not sandwiches.

The Cholera Is Coming!

The impending cholera crisis jolted the rich from their smug self-righteousness. Other epidemic diseases struck mostly the poor, but cholera climbed the social ladder. Both rich and poor died by the thousands. A banker could leave home healthy in the morning and return home that evening in a coffin.

The authorities were panicked. They had ignored Chadwick's warnings. How could they clean up in time to avoid blame for this wave of death? The *Times* wrote of one town:

> The offal [sewage] of a population of eight thousand lies upon the surface of the streets and alleys in its most disgusting form. The only resemblance to a drain is a ditch which surrounds the town, full of black and stagnant matter, and forms the last receptacle for all the carrion that is too bulky and offensive to wither in the streets.[3]

Doctors had treatments from A to Z: Alcohol, Bleeding, Charcoal, Drinking water, cold Effusion, Figs, laughing Gas, Hot tea, Ice, and so on. Lots of ideas, but Chadwick wrote, "All . . . have been employed alike in vain."[4]

The Crisis

When the cholera first invaded, the guilty local officials tried to hide it. But by September 1848, every town knew it was under siege. Cholera first infiltrated the poorest neighborhoods, where generation after generation inherited filth and epidemics. Compared with the 1832 epidemic, the first victim in Leith lived in the same house; in Bermondsey, next to the same open sewer;

in Pollokshaws, the first victim died in the same bed. Nothing had changed. Having ignored Chadwick's sewer solutions, thousands were doomed to death.

Parliament members fled to their country homes. Chadwick knew the danger; he had suffered the cholera twice yet he stayed in London to fight. Day and night he worked to find and flush the sewers and cesspools of London. He hoped that removing the city's sewage might slow the raging epidemic.

Unfortunately London still used the Thames River as both its sewer main and its water main. London's sewers flowed into the Thames above the source for London's drinking water. Thus by flushing out the sewers, Chadwick may have been cleaning the city but he was also flushing the cholera germ into the worst imaginable place—the drinking water of London.

Previously Chadwick had tried to reroute the sewers to clean up the drinking water, but Parliament had ignored his warnings. Now his stopgap method would backfire and make the epidemic even worse.

The London epidemic raged for a full year. In the last cholera epidemic only 16,000 had died; this time over 72,000 died.

Great Man or Great Menace

Chadwick had made a long list of enemies.

The Philosophers

Many felt that the poor were merely victims of fate. Why try to change things? As Chadwick's superior, Lord Seymor, would put it, "There must be poor."[5] Chadwick scorned this convenient "theory that physical degradation and misery were . . . a proper necessity for the great mass of the population."[6]

The Welfare Department

Chadwick had found one orphanage of 1,400 children where 300 had caught cholera and 180 died. The orphanage basement formed a stagnant cesspool for the children's excrement. Orphans, both sick and well, slept three to four in a bed—the well children lying in the diarrhea of the sick. Immediately Chadwick separated the sick from the well. He took fifty men to dig out the filth from the basement. The *Times* reported that many of the orphans were malnourished, potbellied, plastered with impetigo scabs, and infested with scabies. Chadwick had publicly exposed the neglect of the Welfare Department.[7] Now these lazy bureaucrats were out to get Chadwick.

The Treasury Department

While the cholera raged, Chadwick needed more doctors to treat the thousands of victims. In the emergency, he had simply hired doctors without awaiting Treasury approval. Six months after the epidemic let up, the Treasury finally answered his funding request by scolding him for spending funds without official approval.

The Landlords

Landlords objected to Chadwick's "socialism." "What business," they asked, "does the government have with sewers? . . . Let market forces work. . . . People will pay for what they want. . . ." But how well were the market forces working? The *London Gazette* reported:

> the case of a well supplying a dozen houses, which was surrounded by four cesspools within a radius of twelve yards. The water was as thick as soup with seeping matter, and the landlord's agent was obliged to pump for an hour every morning before it ran clear enough for use. Of eighty-five occupants of the houses, twenty-two did not use the well, and all escaped, while forty-six of the remaining sixty-three were attacked by choleraic diarrhœa.[8]

The Parliament

Members of Parliament were elected only by landowners, so they were extremely irritated to have their noses rubbed in the sewage of the nonvoting poor. Even the mention of Chadwick's name in Parliament once produced "a perfect outburst of fury."

A *Times* editorial fumed with an irrational hatred toward Chadwick: "The English people would prefer to take the chance of cholera rather than be bullied into health."[9]

Chadwick had known that all great reformers face great resistance. But he was deeply hurt to realize that few men alive were, "so little loved and so intensely hated."[10]

Sane Sanitation

Chadwick would not give up easily. The epidemic had passed, so he wanted to prevent the next epidemic. Instead of stagnant four-foot tunnels, he found that a four-inch pipe could easily drain the sewage from more than a thousand people. Even the engineers scoffed at such ridiculous "quart into pint" ideas. Yet, if you look in your basement today, you can thank Edwin Chadwick for your house's four-inch (or less) drain.

He surveyed London to devise a sewer system that would efficiently drain the entire city and keep the raw sewage out of the drinking water. The current sewer system was a maze of unplanned tunnels. Some of them had dead ends without any drainage. When workers found and opened one massive sewer, the local sewage official exclaimed, "It is all a mystery."[11]

After taking a year to complete the survey of London, Chadwick began to install a completely new sewer system. By 1853 four-inch pipes were draining more than 27,000 London homes. Towns all over England were installing Chadwick's pipes. In the towns implementing Chadwick's plans, death rates were cut in half. A complete system for England would have saved 150,000 lives every year. The average life expectancy would have jumped from 29 to 48.

The rich and powerful were not impressed. The *Morning Chronicle* declared that Chadwick was making a dung heap out of a speck of dirt. The solution was simple. Just dig a cesspool for every house and dig new drains under the roads. Who needed a bureaucrat "to tell the People of England . . . how each man is to make his drains and [toilets]?"[12] Of course that is exactly what England needed. But Chadwick was a man ahead of his time.

Chadwick's colleague Lord Ashley lamented in his diary, "I do much deplore that our anxieties and labours should be thrown away, and we be told that we have done nothing, attempted nothing, imagined nothing, wished nothing."[13] Ninety-eight years later, Chadwick's first biographer would comment, "Few men have done so much for their fellow-countrymen . . . and received in return so little thanks."[14]

The Ancient Answer

Even without Chadwick's innovations, Europe could have prevented millions of deaths by following directions written thousands of years earlier. With a single sentence, the Bible pointed the way to freedom from deadly epidemics of typhoid, cholera, and dysentery:

> Designate a place outside the camp where you can go to relieve yourself. As part of your equipment have something to dig with, and when you relieve yourself, dig a hole and cover up your excrement.
>
> Deuteronomy 23:12–13 NIV

Used as directed, this one-sentence prescription could have saved more lives than every drug ever made. Compare the prescription with a sentence from a modern camping guide, *Backpacking Basics*. Judge for yourself. Could the biblical writer sue for infringement of patent?

> Go at least 100 yards from water, trails, and camp, somewhere off the beaten path, and dig a hole at least 4 inches deep. To dig, use your heel, a stick, a rock—or a plastic trowel, which I carry for this purpose. . . . Finally, cover the results.[15]

A medical historian writes that the biblical instruction is "an effective [measure] which indicates an advanced idea of sanitation."[16] Short of modern sewage treatment, this may be the best method for disposing of human waste. The biblical method accomplished the most important aspect of public health—separating human waste from human beings. "Careful hygiene," a modern medical textbook states, still "provides the only sure protection against cholera."[17]

Today we understand why God promised, "Obey [this instruction] . . . and I will bring none of these diseases [i.e., typhoid, cholera, dysentery] upon you."

FIVE

A Cemetery Plot

And so, from hour to hour
we ripe and ripe,
And then from hour to
hour we rot and rot,
And thereby hangs a tale.

Shakespeare

If the sanitation of London's living was offensive, the treatment of her dead was positively revolting. A funeral could cost twenty weeks' wages, so a family might struggle for ten or more days to raise the needed funds. Meanwhile, the corpse would be rotting in their home.

Home for most families was a single room. Chadwick noted: "[One room] is their bedroom, their kitchen, their wash-house, their sitting-room, their dining room, and . . . frequently . . . their shop. In this one room they are born, and live, and sleep, and die."[1] Thus, when a relative died, a whole family could live for days in the stench of the rotting corpse. One undertaker noted that families had kept corpses:

. . . even after the coffins had been tapped to let out the liquid products of decomposition, till maggots were seen crawling about the floor . . . till, as the body was borne away, escaping matter ran down the shoulders of the bearers.[2]

It definitely put the pall in pallbearing.

If the person had died of typhus, typhus-carrying lice would leave the cold body to feed on the warm bodies in the room. Four children and a husband might rapidly join a typhus victim in the grave.

When the corpse finally arrived at the cemetery, the situation was no better. A single grave might hold the bodies of eight adults and twenty to thirty children—the whole decomposing heap covered with a thin layer of dirt. When a grave could hold no more, workers made more room by chopping up the bodies with axes. Many bodies were actually exhumed, ground up, and sold to farmers as fertilizer.

One minister described the ground of a cemetery as "saturated and blackened with human remains and fragments of the dead. . . . The splash of water is heard from the graves, as the coffins descend, producing a shudder in every mourner."[3]

With two hundred cemeteries, London's air reeked with the smell of rotting human flesh. Could it be healthy to breathe that everyday smell of London?

The Cemetery Solution

Without extra pay and working sixteen-hour days, Chadwick devised a comprehensive plan to deal with the problem. Parliament must prohibit all burials within the city limits. Churchyards could be planted with grass and used as neighborhood parks. Outside of London, fields would be converted to large cemeteries equipped with chapels and beautiful landscaping. Bodies would no longer lie rotting in people's homes; workers would remove them quickly to mortuaries. There they could be stored for three days before floating up the Thames on funeral barges to the cemeteries.

Of £24,000,000 in bank savings, the English people were earmarking almost 30 percent just for funerals. Chadwick estimated that in London alone nearly one million pounds was "annually thrown into the grave."[4] His plan would cut the cost of burials in half. These savings would in effect create an instant source of wealth for the poor.

Chadwick's ideas upset a lot of coffin carts.

One newspaper found Chadwick's report so disgusting that it refused to report its findings. People hated Chadwick because he refused to sugarcoat reality.

Economists argued that the government should not interfere with the laws of supply and demand. How and where people wanted to be buried was none of the government's business. Chadwick was no savior. He was a tyrant.

Parish priests were upset because they would lose burial fees—a major source of income.

Undertakers were furious. What right did the government have to regulate their profession? Back then, without any formal training, undertakers were merely glorified grave diggers. Charging sky-high fees, London's 3,000-plus undertakers fought for the average 114 weekly funerals. In Chadwick's mind, society would be better off without most of them. Some could work at the new mortuaries and cemeteries; the rest could find other lines of work.

Chadwick Sacked

In the end, Chadwick's plan would neither succeed nor fail; it would simply not be tried. In 1854 Chadwick's direct superior, Lord Seymor, had had enough of Chadwick's activism. Seymor's rule of government was "never to act until he was obliged and then to do as little as he could."[5]

Seymor stood up in Parliament and delivered a blistering speech. He saw Chadwick as an evil power-grabber, violating people's right to bury their relatives as they pleased. As he put it:

All the ordinary feelings of mankind were to be set aside, all the tender emotions of relations to be trampled upon, all the decency of mourning, all the sanctity of grief to be superseded, in order that the Board of Health might get their annual fee.[6]

In the face of this vicious attack, even Chadwick's friends remained silent.

When Chadwick had taken his position on the Board of Health, he had written in his diary: "It will involve trouble, anxiety, reproach, abuse, unpopularity. I shall become a target for private assault and the public Press. . . . God give me strength."[7]

His words had been prophetic. By 1854 the stress left him ill with fever and an upset stomach. Soon the wheels of power would turn and crush him. Parliament was fed up with Chadwick's embarrassing reports, so they simply dissolved the Board of Health and forced Chadwick into early retirement. He had served twenty-two years of ten- to twelve-hour days and had devised plans way ahead of his contemporaries. Today every modern city has enacted virtually every idea that Chadwick devised.

For most of Chadwick's thirty-six years of forced retirement, people universally denounced him. Chadwickism was to the nineteenth century what McCarthyism would be to the twentieth. Just months before Chadwick's death, however, one newspaper finally gave him some due credit: "Had he killed in battle as many as he saved by sanitation, he would have had equestrian statues by the dozen put up to his memory."[8]

Even today, however, historians still confuse the legendary Chadwick, a dogmatic power monger, with the historical Chadwick, the first great sanitary genius.

Before Dusk

For decades England's poor would continue to pass diseases from the dead to the living. Like evil spirits escaping from dead bodies, deadly germs would crawl and drip from the festering coffins and enter the rest of the family.

Yet again, if we rewind the biblical tape, we can hear God giving directions that could have spared thousands of lives. In

Deuteronomy 21:23 God directed the people not to leave even executed criminals unburied. Even murderers, strung up for all to see, were not to be left hanging for days. They were to be buried that same day before dusk.[9]

Much later, when Jesus walked the earth, his close friend Lazarus died. Lazarus's relatives buried him immediately; they didn't even wait for Jesus to arrive. When Jesus did arrive, Martha was horrified that he might open the tomb, because she said, "It's been four days [since he died]; by now he stinks" (John 11:39).[10]

What a different attitude than nineteenth-century England! By insisting on rapid burials, God was not trampling on the "tender emotions of relations" or the "decency of mourning." He was simply desiring the good health of the people.

Buried before sundown, the corpse took its germs with it to the grave; and the people experienced the promise, "none of these diseases . . ."

PART 2

PHYSICAL
WHOLENESS

SIX

Beelzebub in a Bottle

Liquid Lucifer

Give him your self-control,
   and laugh.
Give him your heart,
   and cry.
He takes your will;
   you beg.
He takes your soul. . . .

My (SIM) phone rang about midnight. "Doc, come out here right away! Two people were killed on Route 19. Two others are in bad shape!"

By the time I arrived, a crowd had already gathered. The car had hit a bridge abutment, smashing the steering wheel into the driver's chest. He was obviously dead. The lifeless body of one woman had hurtled thirty feet into a dry creek bed. Another woman lay moaning on the crumpled windshield that she took with her as she flew forward. A semiconscious man lay moaning in the mud.

A shattered whiskey bottle and unbuckled seat belts told of a senseless tragedy.

Devil in the Driver's Seat

Every year almost as many Americans die in their cars as died in the entire twelve-year Vietnam War. Two-thirds of these deaths involve alcohol.[1]

Back in the 1970s, after losing another victim of a drunken driver, an ER doctor asked the attending police officer why he didn't set up roadblocks to catch drunken drivers. The policeman looked at the doctor as though he had just been asked to shoot shoplifters. "We would never do that," he said.

The frustrated doctor pleaded, "Why not? These are people; not roadkill."

Of course this incident did little to help, but the educational efforts of MADD (Mothers Against Drunk Driving) and others have finally changed public attitudes.

No longer is drinking and driving seen as just another part of the normal American lifestyle. Drinking and driving is now treated for what it is—a crime against society and our children.

The Satanic Spirits

I remember the night I (SIM) was called to a nearby home. As I opened my car door, I heard an angry man screaming obscenities and a terrified woman crying for help. Their five frightened children stared desperately out an upstairs window.

I entered the front door to find a drunken husband pressing a handgun to his wife's ear. I reminded him that if he pulled the trigger, he would face the death penalty. I told him that his children would grow up as orphans. I even reminded him how everyone would forget all his fine community work.

Finally, he shoved his wife across the room and cursed her. "If I didn't think I'd hang for this, I'd blow your brains out!"

Unfortunately not every drunk listens to reason. Many commit violent crimes: 53 percent of murders, 57 percent of rapes, 47 percent of robberies, and 60 percent of assaults.[2] Up to 80 percent of suicide victims have allowed alcohol to rob them of their better judgment.[3]

How strange! Free citizens will gleefully take a drug that turns them into violent criminals. The devil himself could not devise a more diabolical scheme.

The Diseases of Drink

Alcohol poisons every organ of the body and causes many diseases:

Nerve Damage

Alcohol poisons nerves. One in five alcoholics develops partial paralysis or permanent pain. One of our patients complained that he couldn't raise his hands high enough to shave his beard. Another complained that every step hurt like a hundred nails jabbing his feet.

Liver Damage

Alcohol poisons the liver. The liver becomes rock hard with cirrhosis. Blood can barely squeeze through. Massive back pressure squeezes fluid out into the legs and abdomen. The belly becomes so distended that the patient struggles even to breathe. We can drain this fluid with a needle, but within weeks or days the fluid usually returns. Despite modern treatments, the fluid accumulates faster and faster.

Blood bypasses the dammed-up liver through other veins, including those in the esophagus (the tube to the stomach). These veins balloon and may rupture. Vomiting buckets of bright red blood, the alcoholic often bleeds to death.

Heart Damage

Alcohol poisons the heart. Over the years it may turn the heart into a big floppy sack that can barely pump blood. The legs and abdomen swell up with backed-up fluid. Without warning the heart may slip into a spastic rhythm, causing sudden death.

Brain Damage

Alcohol and its related vitamin deficiencies poison the brain. The alcoholic may lose his memory and make up wild stories to fill in the gaps. He can't find his keys, so his brain fills the gap with a story of thieves stealing them. He forgot that he left the front door open, so he imagines that aliens must have entered his house. It may sound funny, but it is a tragedy for his loved ones.

Withdrawal Agonies

As an intern, I (SIM) saw a man, who was suffering alcohol withdrawal, ride into the hospital ward on a pink elephant. At least he *thought* he was riding one. Another screamed as a pack of scarlet gorillas was tearing him apart. Bedlam erupted in the large wards of that day as patients shouted at and hid from imaginary beasts.

Once I saw a patient smash a twentieth-story window to leap from his hallucination. Fortunately a nurse caught the tail of his gown and pulled him back. We had to handcuff these patients to their beds and give them large doses of morphine, but even with our best treatments many of them died.

In today's hospitals, medications control most withdrawal symptoms. In the community, however, many alcoholics keep drinking just to avoid the terrors of withdrawal.

Damage to the Unborn

When a mother drinks, her unborn baby also drinks, as alcohol passes freely from mother to fetus. The baby may become an alcoholic while still inside the mother. At birth these babies must endure the agonies of alcohol withdrawal for several days in the neonatal intensive care unit.

Babies born to drinkers are prone to mental retardation, poor coordination, and abnormal brain waves—the fetal alcohol syndrome. Even the casual-drinking mother risks miscarriage, premature delivery, and a handicapped child. It takes so little alcohol to cause some of this damage that doctors now warn mothers not to drink any alcohol at any time during pregnancy.

Sexual Disorders

In popular myth, alcohol boosts sexual potency. In reality, alcoholics suffer lower testosterone levels and impaired sexual function and drive. They were the first in line to try Viagra. Shakespeare observed : Drink "provokes the desire, but it takes away the performance."[4]

The King of Tears

TV ads, neon signs, and social parties try to blind us to alcohol's destructive force. Doctors, however, cannot hide from the reality, for alcohol's victims are our patients.

One day a forty-two-year-old man visited my (DES) office with his mother. George's skin shone bright yellow. He staggered from the chair to the exam table. George wanted relief from his severe abdominal pain.

He lived with his mother, who confirmed that he had not eaten a single bite of food for over fourteen months. Every day, he took in over 3,000 calories in beer. "That," she said, "is not a balanced diet." I agreed. I didn't even know that it was possible to live that long on beer alone.

He was suffering from a massively swollen, tender liver. The yellow jaundice came from a backup of bile. His staggering gait was from nerve damage; he couldn't even feel his feet.

George refused hospitalization. He refused to stop drinking but he would "try to cut back." He knew that he was near death but all he wanted was pain medicine. I refused. Pain was his only hope. Pain was the only thing that might force him to get help and dry out.

His mother pleaded with him. But his common sense had long since dissolved in beer. He thanked me for my concern; but if I still refused pain pills, he would just go back home.

I tried to get the courts to intervene, but they said we had to wait until he was no longer "competent to make his own decisions."

Four weeks later he slipped into a coma. His mother called an ambulance. In the hospital he awoke. Medications blocked withdrawal symptoms, and his liver slowly recovered. He received thousands of dollars of counseling and hospitalization.

When he got back home, his first act was to drink a six-pack of beer. Maybe the so-called King of Beers might be better called The King of Tears.

> I drank for happiness,
>   and became unhappy.
> I drank for joy,
>   and became miserable.
> I drank for sociability,
>   and became argumentative.
> I drank for sophistication,
>   and became obnoxious.
> I drank for friendship,
>   and made enemies.
> I drank for sleep,
>   and woke up tired.
> I drank for strength,
>   and felt weak.
> I drank for relaxation,
>   and got the shakes.
> I drank for courage,
>   and became afraid.
> I drank for confidence,
>   and became doubtful.
> I drank for conversation,
>   and slurred my speech.
> I drank to feel heavenly,
>   and ended up feeling like hell.
>   author unknown

Licensed Larceny

Shakespeare marveled in *Macbeth*, "O God! That men should put an enemy in their mouths to steal away their brains. . . ." But alcohol not only robs their brains, it strips them of their health and their children's health. It even picks their pockets. Money that should provide a family with food, clothes, and housing is far too often tossed over the bar, damning a family to poverty, neglect, and sickness.

Accident prone, the alcoholic wanders through the workday like a car veering through a dense fog. He causes almost half of the annual five thousand work-related deaths.

Some defend this massacre by pointing out that alcohol gives back to society. Alcohol pays billions in taxes. Alcohol ads fund hundreds of TV football games. Alcohol creates thousands of jobs: farmers, bartenders, doctors, policemen, and undertakers.

Sure, alcohol provides jobs, but what does alcohol take in return?

- thousands of highway deaths
- thousands of murder victims
- thousands of sickly people
- thousands of broken marriages
- thousands of fatherless children

Alcohol's slogan might be, "Jobs for lives." Sounds like a bargain—a bargain with the devil.

Even on a strictly net financial basis, alcohol robs American society of hundreds of billions of dollars. Costs resulting from alcohol make up 10 percent of your health insurance and 40 percent of your auto insurance premium. Alcohol abuse costs society more than every cancer and every lung disease combined.[5]

Think of a class of forty first-graders. Then put a red X over two of their faces. If we do nothing, two of them (on average) will die from alcohol.

God's Warnings

Living by the Bible immunizes us to the tragedies of alcohol. The Bible clearly says:

> Don't be a fool;
>> Realize that God doesn't want you,
>> To waste your life,
>> Drunk on alcoholic spirits.
> Instead be filled with the Holy Spirit.
>> Ephesians 5:17–18

One Scripture warns in crisp, colorful language of the economic, medical, and social ravages of alcohol. It even describes the hallucinations of alcohol withdrawal.

> Listen, my son, and be wise,
>> be guided by good sense:
> never sit down with tipsy men
>> or among gluttons;
> the drunkard and the glutton come to poverty,
>> and revelling leaves men in rags.
>
> Who shriek? Who groan?
>> Who quarrel and grumble?
> Who are bruised for nothing?
>> Who have bleary eyes?
> Those who linger over the bottle,
>> those who relish blended wines.
> Then look not on the wine so red,
>> that sparkles in the cup;
> it glides down smoothly at the first,
>> but in the end it bites like any snake,
> it stings you like an adder.
>> You will be seeing odd things,
>> you will be saying queer things;
> you will be like a man asleep at sea,
>> asleep in the midst of a storm.
>> Proverbs 23:19–21, 29–34 Moffatt

Bill W.

Many a man and woman have ignored these plain Scriptures and skipped lightly down the alcohol road, reaching its dead end: imprisoned for umpteen DWIs, divorced by their only human love, penniless on skid row, or in a thousand other tragic circumstances.

For the entire twentieth century, doctors examined, treated, and studied alcoholics. They applied the latest psychological theories. They infused the latest drugs. No matter what they tried, they had the same result—failure. Even the medical community has realized that a purely medical approach to alcoholism is next to worthless.

Bill W. had discovered this. He had once been a successful Wall Street investor. Now he struggled to even pay the rent. Malnutrition left him forty pounds underweight.

At his third hospitalization to dry out, a doctor explained that alcoholics have a weakness. In other areas, alcoholics may be tree trunks of willpower, but when it comes to alcohol their willpower is flimsier than a blade of grass.

Now Bill had a grasp on his problem; he must stay alert and strengthen his willpower. Later he wrote: "Understanding myself now, I fared forth in high hope. For three or four months the goose hung high. I went to town regularly and even made a little money. Surely this was the answer—self-knowledge. But it was not, for the frightful day came when I drank once more."[6]

His health began to fail. Doctors told his wife he would likely be dead or institutionalized within a year. He gave up hope but not alcohol. One day Bill's old friend Ebby phoned. Bill was relieved; the rumors that the courts had committed Ebby to a mental institution were false.

Ebby was a great drinker. Once Bill and Ebby had even chartered an airplane to finish a drinking spree. As Bill sat at the restaurant table, he looked forward to drinking and reminiscing. He was in for a surprise.

The door opened and he [Ebby] stood there, fresh-skinned and glowing. There was something about his eyes. He was inexplicably different. What had happened? I pushed a drink across the table. He refused it. . . . He wasn't himself. "Come, what's all this about?" I queried. . . .

Smilingly, he said, "I've got religion." I was aghast. So that was it—last summer an alcoholic crackpot; now, I suspected, a little cracked about religion.[7]

Bill considered religion useless: "With ministers, and the world's religions, I parted right there. When they talked of a God personal to me, . . . I became irritated and my mind snapped shut against such a theory."[8]

Ebby's sobriety, however, could not be so easily dismissed. "His human will had failed. Doctors had pronounced him incurable. Society was about to lock him up. . . . God had done for him what he could not do for himself."[9] God had changed him from the inside out. Ebby suggested that Bill start with what he could believe about God and move from there.[10]

Ebby took Bill to Calvary Rescue Mission, where Rev. Sam Shoemaker preached the five Cs for experiencing Christ's power to save:[11]

- **Confidence:** Ebby had shared his own sins and failures in *confidence* with Bill.
- **Confession:** Ebby encouraged Bill to *confess* his own sins and failures.
- **Conviction:** Ebby had to draw Bill into a *conviction* of his sins and an awareness that Christ was the answer for them.
- **Conversion:** Bill would be born again when he gave himself to God and confessed Jesus as Lord and that God raised him from the dead.[12]
- **Continuance:** Bill needed to *continue* in personal prayer, Bible study, church attendance, and sharing with others what God had done for him.[13]

At one meeting Bill "humbly offered [himself] to God." At that moment, "For sure," he later wrote, "I'd been born again."[14]

He signed himself back into the hospital, dried out, and was released. He worked hard to apply Rev. Sam's teachings. He admitted that he was hopeless and needed God. Years later Bill wrote:

> I placed myself unreservedly under [God's] care and direction. I admitted for the first time that of myself I was nothing; that without Him I was lost. I ruthlessly faced my sins. . . .
>
> We made a list of people I had hurt or toward whom I felt resentment. . . . I was to right all such matters to the utmost of my ability. . . .[15]

Rev. Sam taught Bill that owning up to one's sins, "is not the mark of a sick soul, but rather the sign of return to spiritual health."[16] If Bill was serious about dealing with his sin, he must "face it, share it, surrender it. Hate it, forsake it, confess it, and restore for it."[17]

Bill never again tasted Demon Rum. He joined with others who had the same saving experience, and they started sharing the good news with thousands. They stressed the basics of Christianity: "God, the Bible, prayer, Quiet Time, surrenders to God (actually acceptance of Jesus Christ as Savior), Christian literature, Christian fellowship, and daily Bible devotionals."[18]

They established a program to help alcoholics. In it an alcoholic was required to spend one week in the hospital drying out. In the hospital room, Bill and his colleagues allowed only one book—the Bible.

The results amazed everyone. An astounding 50 percent of "medically incurable" alcoholics who "really tried" stayed sober. Another 25 percent sobered up after a few relapses. No one, before or since, has seen such results.

Advice to a Young Sot
Leave Beelzebub in his bottle;
Take God out of your box.

Bill's group grew into the worldwide organization, Alcoholics Anonymous. Bill gave credit for the entire "spiritual substance" of steps three through twelve[19] "directly to [Rev.] Samuel Shoe-maker."[20] Where did Rev. Sam get them? The Bible.

Today A.A. has strayed from its distinctly Christian roots, and its results have become much less impressive.[21] Even so, this worldwide organization has used basic biblical principles to help millions of alcoholics get and stay sober. Almost all medical and psychological programs use A.A. as part of their therapy.

The *Big Book* of Alcoholics Anonymous states that only God is the answer:

> We [alcoholics] had to fearlessly face the proposition that . . . God either is, or He isn't. . . .
>
> If you think you are an atheist, an agnostic, a skeptic, or have any other form of intellectual pride which keeps you from accepting [A.A.]. . . I feel sorry for you. . . .
>
> We have an answer for you. It never fails, if you go about it with one-half the zeal you have been in the habit of showing when you were getting another drink. Your heavenly Father will never let you down!
>
> There is One who has all power—that One is God. May you find Him now![22]

Rev. Sam spoke clearly:

> Willpower, and the appeal to it as sufficient to get any of us out of [our] troubles, [is] a snare and a delusion. . . . When you think you're able to manage your life without God, you add pride to whatever other sins you may have. . . .[23]
>
> What you want is simply a vital religious experience. You need to find God. You need Jesus Christ.[24]

If God is left out, all programs to reform the alcoholic will fail. Medicine cannot cure. Psychology cannot transform. Self-help books cannot help.

An alcoholic needs God.

SEVEN

Cancer by the Carton

Tobacco is a filthy weed;
That from the Devil does
    proceed.
It drains your purse;
It burns your clothes;
and makes a chimney of
    your nose.

Benjamin Waterhouse,
1754–1846,
founding professor,
Harvard Medical School

The local grocery store manager phoned me (SIM) one day. "Doctor," he said, "Mrs. Henderson slipped me a note this morning when I delivered groceries to her house. Her husband is very sick. He won't let her leave the house for fear she will never come back. She's afraid he may kill her. She wants you to go over to her house."

I was amazed at the change in Mr. Henderson. He had been a tall, muscular ex-footballer. Now with his flesh wasted away and his eyes sunken, he looked more like a prisoner from Auschwitz. Coughing up clots of blood, he had not slept well for months.

We were all relieved when he finally consented to hospital admission. His first night in the hospital, however, he suffered massive lung bleeding and drowned, gurgling in his own blood.

An autopsy revealed a massive lung cancer that had spread to his ribs, pelvis, liver, neck, and brain.

The Lung Cancer Epidemic

In 1912 a medical text called lung cancer "the rarest of diseases."[1] What a change a century can make! Today lung cancer is America's number one cancer killer, causing one in four cancer deaths. Annually lung cancer chokes the life out of 120,000 Americans; that's over 300 funerals every day.

What caused this lung cancer epidemic? Was it air pollution? No, air pollution causes less than 5 percent of lung cancers.[2] Was it radon? No, radon causes only a small fraction of cases. Was it food additives? No. Was it pesticides? No. None of these factors have made a detectable change in the rate of any major cancer.

When the statistics shot up, many doctors suspected the cause, but proof did not come until 1950. Drs. Wynder and Graham reported 605 consecutive proven lung cancer victims: 597 were smokers; only 8 were nonsmokers. Since then, thousands of studies have proven that smoking is the only major cause of lung cancer.

The more you smoke, the more risk you take. Half-pack-a-day smokers suffer more heart attacks and cancers. Heavy smokers suffer up to 34 times more laryngeal (voice box) cancer and 72 times more lung cancer.

Smoking causes cancers of the bladder, pancreas, and breast. How can smoking cause cancer in organs that never directly contact smoke? Cigarette smoke contains more than forty cancer-causing chemicals. In the lung, these chemicals rapidly dissolve in the blood and flow out to poison every organ in the body.

Toxins in cigarette smoke include carbon monoxide, ammonia, cyanide, acetone, benzene, phenol, DDT, methanol, arsenic, formaldehyde, nitrobenzene, ammonia, hydrogen cyanide, and a radioactive element polonium-210. This partial list shows that a smoker uses his body as a toxic-waste dump, rivaling even Love Canal.

The Heart Connection

Once I (SIM) was called out of bed to treat a forty-two-year-old man, stricken with sudden, crushing chest pain. When I arrived, the man lay ashen gray on the floor. His eyes stared blankly at the ceiling. He was not breathing. He had no pulse. He was dead. A clot in a coronary artery had shut off the blood supply to his heart, changing this muscular pump into a lifeless sack.

A pack of cigarettes tucked into his shirt pocket explained why he had suffered a fatal heart attack at such an early age. Cigarettes kill more than 200,000 Americans every year by heart attack.

A pack of cigarettes is a fistful of coffin nails. Heavy smokers shorten their lives by an average of eight years. On average, *every cigarette* smoked shortens a life by about *five minutes*. Cigarette smoke causes narrowed arteries and stickier blood cells. The thickened blood tends to clot in the narrowed coronary arteries, and suddenly, a heart attack.

Compared with the nonsmoker's, the smoker's heart attack is generally more serious. Carbon monoxide has depleted oxygen from his blood, but his nicotine-stimulated heart needs even more oxygen. With oxygen supply down and oxygen demand up, the smoker's heart attack kills more heart cells and is more likely to kill him.

Tobacco-damaged arteries harm other body parts. In the brain, they cause strokes. In the legs, they cause gangrene. A damaged aorta may swell up and rupture. Most victims of these ruptured aneurysms die without making it to the operating room.

Tobacco companies responded to these health alarms by manufacturing so-called low tar cigarettes. They used lasers to perforate the cigarette paper, so that the government test machines would suck in outside air and register lower tar and nicotine levels. Unfortunately for smokers, these holes were strategically placed so that the smoker's lips and fingers would block them. Thus, in actual smokers, the labeled "tar and nicotine content" does not accurately indicate the consumed levels of carbon monoxide or nicotine.[3]

Whether one smokes "low tar" or "high tar" cigarettes, the heart attack risk remains the same. The number, not the type, of cigarettes determines the heart attack risk. Thus the "low risk" cigarette does not exist.[4]

Actually it does exist; you just can't buy it. Back in the 1970s one company did spend over ten million dollars and patented a cigarette, eliminating many harmful chemicals. Studies found that these cigarettes caused much less cancer in mice. But they decided not to market it. Their lawyers warned them that marketing a safer cigarette meant admitting the other cigarettes were not safe. Their need to perpetuate their lie kept a safer cigarette out of the hands of the nicotine addicts it may have benefited.[5]

Emphysema

In the lungs, a spring-like protein, elastin, forms a suspension system that keeps the tiny air tubules expanded. Smoking causes enzymes to break down elastin and smoking blocks the body's ability to repair this breakdown. The lung's elastic suspension disintegrates, and the tubules collapse. Over several years, the smoker slowly suffocates.

One of my (DES) patients had such severe emphysema that he could not even dress himself without becoming breathless. A tube supplied continuous oxygen through a hole in his neck. Unable to completely exhale through his collapsed airways, air got trapped in his lungs. His chest overinflated until it assumed the shape of a pickle barrel. For seven years, his activity was limited to rolling over in bed, changing TV channels, and smoking his demon cigarettes through the hole in his neck. The Veterans Administration hospital where he stayed housed twenty other permanent lung invalids.

Wrinkled and Sterile

Smoking poisons the skin, causing the wrinkled raisin look, so common in elderly smokers.[6] Americans seem almost schizophrenic. They spend billions of dollars to try to look better. Every year they turn right around and spend over forty billion dollars on cigarettes to destroy those looks.

Smoking also causes male infertility. Male smokers have lower sperm counts. What sperm they have are deformed and sluggish. Tell that to the next teenage boy who thinks smoking is macho.

The Woman Killer

In 1900 less than 6 percent of women smoked. By 1999, 22 percent of women had picked up the habit, and the epidemic of women smokers continues to worsen. During the 1990s, the number of teenage girls who smoke shot up by 33 percent.[7]

But tobacco is not sexist; it is just as happy to kill a woman as a man. From 1960 to 1999 lung cancer deaths in women increased by 400 percent. It has even surpassed breast cancer as the number one cancer-killer in women. Women truly have "come a long way, baby."

Despite the evidence, for over fifty years the tobacco companies have continued to deny the risk. One tobacco CEO stated under oath in 1994, "We have looked . . . at all the statistical data [and] that has not convinced me that smoking causes death."[8]

Secondhand Sickness

Ryan's mother was frustrated. "Why is Ryan always sick? Doctors don't seem to help."

She had just spent another whole night up with her screaming two year old. In his short life he had already suffered fourteen ear infections and umpteen colds.

The smell of his clothes suggested the cause of his suffering. "Sarah," I (DES) said, "you need to stop smoking. It's poisoning his body."

"Oh, yeah," she said. "It's my only bad habit. . . . I think he has allergies. . . . Would taking a vitamin help?"

I told her the proven dangers of secondhand smoke, especially to children. I told her that spending one hour in a smoky room is the equivalent of smoking one cigarette.[9] Ryan was smoking the equivalent of half a pack daily.

No matter what I said, Sarah wouldn't listen. Her nicotine addiction was so strong that she wouldn't even think about quitting for her son's health. She kept smoking, and I saw Ryan back for many more illnesses over the next few years.

Every day millions of babies breathe into their fragile lungs smoke from their parents' cigarettes. This sidestream smoke causes 300,000 cases of pneumonia and bronchitis in children every year.[10]

Quit for Fido
Dogs living with smokers
suffer more lung cancer.

Completely unfiltered, sidestream smoke is even more toxic than mainstream smoke. Sidestream smoke contains higher concentrations of over thirty-nine toxic chemicals. One extremely potent cancer-causing chemical, dimethylnitrosamine, is up to 830 times more concentrated in sidestream smoke.

Women married to smokers have higher rates of lung cancer. The CDC estimates that in the United States, secondhand smoke causes 3,000 deaths every year.[11]

Harming the Unborn

Children of mothers who smoked during pregnancy are (on average) shorter, sicker, and less intelligent than children of mothers who didn't smoke. By age eleven these children average an inch shorter and lag six months behind their peers in reading and math. These handicaps are even seen in children whose mothers smoked less than half a pack daily.[12]

Smoking mothers have twice as many stillbirths.[13] Their liveborn babies are smaller and more likely to suffer complications and die.[14]

Sometimes seemingly healthy babies suddenly die without any explanation. This Sudden Infant Death Syndrome (SIDS) leaves families devastated and wondering, "Why us?" One reason is smoking. Secondhand smoke doubles the risk for SIDS. If the mother also smoked while pregnant, the SIDS risk triples.[15] Keeping smoke away from babies is truly a matter of life and death.

Tobacco for Teens

Most efforts to curtail smoking focus on education, and the education has worked. Today almost all teens know that smoking is harmful. Still, one in five high school seniors smokes.[16] Even college students are smoking in record numbers, their numbers increasing by 28 percent from 1993 to 1997.[17]

3000
Number of teens in the United States
who start smoking every day
1000
Number of those teens who will die
of a smoking-related disease

Since over 80 percent of smokers start before their sixteenth birthday, the tobacco cartel knows they must get their victims young. Sales representatives for Big Tobacco focus on the so-called young adult market by plastering extra ads in stores and on billboards near high schools and colleges.[18]

They have even directed their campaigns at young children and these campaigns have worked. In the 1990s, 91 percent of six year olds could match up Joe Camel with a cigarette. The tobacco kings grinned; they knew that these kids would grow up into a bumper crop of teen smokers.

Our Boys and Why They Should Not Smoke
Many a man smokes one or two hundred pounds worth
of tobacco during the best part of his life; after all, what
has he got for it? A damaged constitution, a horrible
breath, and a constant craving for another smoke.

British Anti-Tobacco and Anti-Narcotic League pamphlet,
c. 1900[19]

King Tobacco has spent billions to promote the sexy, macho cigarette image. Researchers suspected it had altered the perceptions of teens, so they did a simple experiment. They asked teens to describe two nearly identical pictures of a man, one with a cigarette and one without. Teens tended to describe the smoker as adventurous, rugged, daring, and energetic. They tended to describe the nonsmoker as shy, gentle, and awkward.[20] The macho Marlboro men and the sexy Salem beauties have convinced today's teens that smoking is cool, fun, and mature.

Sure, they know smoking is dangerous, but teens desperately want to feel grown up. King Tobacco knows this. That's why almost every issue of *Teen* and *Young Miss* has carried an ad from R. J. Reynolds urging kids not to smoke. But the ads don't tell them to refrain because it is addictive or it might kill them. No, they tell the teens to wait because the choice to smoke is an "adult decision." Another brochure, "Tobacco: Helping Youth Say No," doesn't mention any of tobacco's dangers. Parents are to tell their children that adults smoke because "they enjoy it."[21]

What a brilliant deception! "Don't do it. It's really fun, but it's just for grown ups. You don't want to have fun and feel grown-up, do you?"

It may look like anti-smoking literature, but it will sell lots of cigarettes.

King Tobacco is happy to let the educators have teenage minds; King Tobacco wants only their hearts.

What to Do

In the seventeenth century, Turks caught smoking were beheaded, hanged, and quartered. The first Russian Czar had smokers castrated, flogged, and exiled to Siberia. That's a bit much, but less severe measures can make a big difference.

Tax, Tax, Tax

The quickest way to reduce smoking is to increase the price of a pack of cigarettes. Many studies have shown that when cigarette prices go up, sales go down. It's only fair to tax smokers to help cover their excessive consumption of health-care dollars.

Make Big Tobacco Pay

For years the tobacco giants have spent billions of dollars to deceive the public about the dangers of tobacco. They have even paid scientists to falsely debunk the studies of tobacco's dangers. As late as 1994, the CEO of R. J. Reynolds stated under oath, "Smoking is no more addictive than coffee, tea, or Twinkies."[22] The CEO of Brown and Williamson also testified, "I believe nicotine is not addictive."[23] Since then a secret document has come to light. Thirty years earlier, his own company lawyer had noted, "We are, then, in the business of selling nicotine, an addictive drug."[24]

As the massive scale of Big Tobacco's deception has become clear, the tobacco giants are beginning to ante up. With a 368-billion-dollar agreement in 1998, they will partially reimburse the states for their excess Medicare costs.

What about the individual victims and their families? Big Tobacco has not paid a penny to them. An army of lawyers has legally blocked compensation to widows and orphans for the wrongful deaths of their loved ones. This is not justice. Big Tobacco must pay for its cigarette seduction.

Ban Advertising

On 13 May 1998 the European Parliament placed a near total ban on tobacco advertising. They banned tobacco ads from billboards, newspapers, and magazines. Sporting event sponsorships are banned. Even logo shirts are banned.

The United States could learn from Europe. Even when Congress banned television ads in the United States, they actually were doing a favor to Big Tobacco. The tobacco cartel wanted to get rid of the Fairness Doctrine, the policy requiring that for every pro-smoking ad on TV, the TV station had to donate one anti-smoking ad. Tobacco ads were stimulating annual sales by seventy-five cigarettes per person, but anti-tobacco ads were cutting sales by an estimated five hundred cigarettes per person.[25] You don't need an MBA to realize that this may have been good for health but it was bad for business.

Big Tobacco desperately wanted the Fairness Doctrine repealed. In exchange cigarette companies would give up TV ads. The deal was cut, and TV cigarette ads disappeared. Without the free ad time, anti-smoking groups no longer had the TV time to tell America the tobacco truth.

Big Tobacco put their TV megabucks into billboards, shirts, race cars, and magazines. Here they met no Fairness Doctrine. Soon they had what they wanted: millions more nicotine addicts.

Big Tobacco was even happy to let the Surgeon General print warnings on every pack. Why? Simple; they hoped the health warnings would protect them from lawsuits by tobacco victims. Victims might sue, but Big Tobacco could answer, "Don't say we didn't warn you." All the while, they could go on denying that cigarettes harm anyone, because it wasn't their warning; it was the Surgeon General's. Big Tobacco has used those warnings to avoid billions of dollars in legal fees and wrongful death payments.

Big Tobacco even controls the information that you read. The few times *Time* magazine has run an article about tobacco's dangers, Big Tobacco has pulled advertising from the next issue, costing *Time* about a million dollars in lost revenue. That is why most magazines no longer print today's news about the dangers of smoking and Big Tobacco's demonic deceptions.

A few brave magazines, including *Readers Digest* and *Saturday Evening Post,* refuse cigarette ads. No wonder these magazines are also among the few who print the truth about tobacco.

Maybe we can't ban tobacco, but surely we can ban Big Tobacco from plastering sexy models and macho cowboys with cigarettes in every magazine and on billboards across the land. Why allow Big Tobacco to seduce one more teen to an early grave?

In stores, cigarettes should be kept out of sight and under the counter. Shiny gold wrappers and T-shirt giveaways should be banned. All brands should be packaged in white wrappers with only plain black lettering allowed. Cigarette vending machines should be banned. The Surgeon General's warning should cover the back of every pack.

We may not ban tobacco but we must not allow these pushers of puff to make their poison so appealing.

Why Do People Smoke?

Parental Examples

The number one factor influencing teens to smoke is parental example. By smoking, parents double the chances that their children will smoke.[26] It may seem crazy, but when kids rebel against their parents, they often simply imitate their parents.

Several studies indicate that parental *attitudes* have *no influence* on whether their children take up the smoking habit.[27] Parents, make sure your actions aren't earplugs in your children's ears. It's what you *do,* not what you say, that counts.

To Look Mature

Many teens see smoking as the gateway to adulthood. It serves as a status symbol to show the world that they have arrived. Smoking soon becomes a social aid. Instead of fidgeting, they have something to do with their hands. Sharing and bumming cigarettes allows them to feel like they belong.

Withdrawal

Every time a smoker's nicotine level drops, he begins to suffer withdrawal symptoms of anxiety and irritation. Seven seconds after inhaling, nicotine rushes to the smoker's brain and relieves the withdrawal anxiety. That is why so many smokers think that smoking relaxes them.

Stress

Stress acidifies the urine and speeds up nicotine excretion. Thus when a person is stressed, he must smoke even more to maintain the same nicotine levels.

Habit

We are creatures of habit. Anything that we repeat every day, we soon do without thinking. Marcel Proust observed that the more absurd a habit, the stronger it is. What could be more absurd than inhaling toxic fumes into delicate lungs?

Addiction

Smoking is as dangerous as any bear trap. Big Tobacco baits the trap with slick advertising and fancy packaging. Teens look at the enticing bait and figure it won't hurt them. After all, they can get out whenever they want. But within a few weeks, the trap jaws of addiction have snapped shut. Any escape will be very painful. Nicotine, pure and simple, is an addictive drug.

In 1980 Philip Morris hired two scientists, Victor DeNoble and Paul Mele, to do addiction studies, using nicotine and rats. They did their work in absolute secrecy, even from fellow Philip Morris scientists. Quickly they found that their rats became heavily addicted and gave themselves bigger-and-bigger nicotine fixes.

One day without warning, DeNoble and Mele were fired. They were ordered to stop their studies immediately, turn off their instruments, and turn in their security badges. According to DeNoble, "The lab literally vanished overnight. The animals were killed, the equipment was removed, and all traces of the former lab were eliminated."[28] Philip Morris even threatened to sue if they discussed or published their research. DeNoble said that Philip Morris executives had correctly understood this research. In terms of addictiveness, "nicotine looked like heroin."[29]

When it comes to nicotine, what's true for mice is true for people. Even smokers who get throat cancer, have their voice box surgically removed, and must breathe and smoke through a hole in the windpipe—even half of these patients go back to smoking. One of our patients smoked three packs of cigarettes a day. At night he even woke up almost every hour to smoke a cigarette.

Sigmund Freud was another nicotine slave. Smoking twenty cigars a day, he suffered forty years of heart disease and endured thirty-three operations for mouth cancer that eventually killed him. His doctors warned him to stop smoking, yet he could not stir up the courage to quit.

The few short times he tried to quit, he found himself miserable with withdrawal. Once when a doctor ordered him to quit, he shot back, "[Would you rather I] have a long miserable life?"[30]

Quitting

Because smoking is such a strong addiction, quitting is never easy. But quitting smoking has tremendous benefits. Within three weeks, young adults have decreased heart rates, more efficient breathing, more elastic lungs, and increased stamina.[31]

Given a deadly diagnosis, some patients finally do quit. But doesn't it make a lot more sense to quit before developing a fatal disease? After only one smoke-free year, you can cut your risk of heart disease in half. After ten years, you cut your risk of lung cancer in half.[32]

Using nicotine patches, inhalers, and medications, today's doctors can help many people who have failed before in their efforts to quit. In my (DES) practice last year, I treated over two hundred smokers for nicotine addiction. About 80 percent were smoke-free at one month. They felt better. They smelled better. They had more energy. They were proud of their achievement.

Doctors Finally Wake Up

I (SIM) once asked another doctor, who had quit smoking, if he had found it difficult. "No," he said, "not after I really made up my mind. When I quit, I got rid of the biggest nuisance in my life."

"What do you mean?" I asked. "I thought people smoked because they enjoyed it."

"It's not like that at all," he replied. "I got rid of a grand nuisance. I was always looking for cigarettes, for matches, for ashtrays. I burned holes in my suits and the furniture. When I quit, I got rid of the biggest annoyance anybody can ever have."

He is only one of thousands of physicians who woke up and smelled the smoke. Years ago at medical meetings, I had to struggle to see the speaker through the smoky haze. For a day or two afterward I smelled like something smoked. Even the *Journal of the American Medical Association* carried ads for cigarettes. In 1949 an incredible 60 percent of physicians smoked.[33] Today only 3 percent smoke.[34]

These drastic changes in doctors' habits occurred when doctors finally realized that smoking is the greatest preventable cause of:

- Health Enemy #1: Heart Disease
- Health Enemy #2: Cancer

All told, cigarettes kill more than 400,000 Americans each year. That is more than all the combined deaths from automobile accidents, AIDS, alcohol, illegal drugs, murder, suicide, and fires.

Point

Have you not reason to be ashamed, and to forbeare this filthie noveltie? . . . In your abuse thereof . . . sinning against God, harming your selves both in persons and goods, . . . [and] making yourselves . . . to be scorned and contemned.

[Smoking is] lothesome to the eye, hatefull to the Nose, harmfull to the braine, dangerous to the Lungs, and the blacke stinking fume thereof, neerest resembling the horrible Stigian smoke of the pit that is bottomlesse.

King James I of England,
A Counterblaste to Tobacco, 1604

Counterpoint

There can be no doubt that tobacco can cleanse all impurities and disperse every gross and viscious humour, as we find by daily experience.

It cures cancer of the breast, open and eating sores scabs and scratches, however poisonous and septic, goitre, broken limbs, erysipelas, and many other things. It will heal wounds in the arms, legs and other members of the body, of however long-standing.

Dr. Johannes Vittich,
respected physician, early 1600s[35]

We Should Have Known

We can be thankful that medical science has opened our eyes to the dangers of smoking. But we can be even more thankful to God for sparing millions of his followers from these horrible diseases. Before any lung cancer studies, before any population surveys, before any Surgeon General reports—God led many to avoid and condemn tobacco.

In 1653 Jacob Bald, a Jesuit priest, asked, "What difference is there between a smoker and a suicide; except that the one takes longer to kill himself than the other?"[36]

That same year, a group of bishops and university professors issued a manifesto stating:

> It is both godless and unseemly that the mouth of man, which is the means of entrance and exit for the immortal soul, that mouth which is intended to breathe in the fresh air and to utter the praises of the Most High, should be defiled by the indrawing and expelling of tobacco smoke.[37]

Throughout the 1800s the temperance movement convinced many Christians to condemn tobacco. In 1881 temperance advocate Frances Willard pledged:

> From all tobacco I'll abstain,
> And never take God's name in vain.[38]

Around 1900 a pamphlet of the British Anti-Tobacco and Anti-Narcotic League exhorted:

> May those who read this paper resolve that they will seek to realize the chief end of their being, which is to glorify God, and to love and imitate the Saviour, and that they will have nothing to do with habits so offensive and injurious as the smoking of Tobacco.[39]

Years ago I (SIM) heard an ex-smoker give testimony. He had been converted in a church where no one preached against smoking, yet the Holy Spirit prompted him to quit. It seemed an odd request, but he obeyed. Sometime later he came across Scriptures that confirmed his leading.

Tobacco was unknown in biblical cultures, so it is no surprise that the Bible doesn't mention it by name. Christians, however, observed tobacco's smells, spittoons, smokes, and sicknesses. They realized that indulgence in tobacco ran contrary to many Bible passages, such as:

> Don't you realize that your body is a temple of the Holy Spirit, who lives in you? . . . You don't own yourself; God bought you at a price. Therefore honor God with your body (1 Cor. 6:19–20).

> God's temple is a holy place, and your body is that temple (1 Cor. 3:17).

> No matter what you are doing, even eating or drinking, do it all for the glory of God (1 Cor. 10:31).

In many religions—such as Hinduism, Shintoism, Buddhism, Gnosticism, and Zoroastrianism—what you do with your body doesn't matter.[40] Only the spiritual is important. But here Christianity parts ways. What you do with your body matters to God. Obedience to this biblical view has spared many Christians. They have had none of these smokes, none of these chews, and "none of these diseases."

EIGHT

Torture or Nurture?

The data . . . have influenced me to change my mind so that I now recommend routine [newborn circumcision]. . . . I no longer believe circumcision is a dirty word; it is clean.

Dr. Thomas Wiswell, 1992

Some say it causes "long-lasting psychological damage to the child."[1] It has been called "child abuse,"[2] "pure and simple torture,"[3] and even "partial castration."[4] What is this "barbaric custom?"[5] Why do over 85 percent of boys undergo it? Why is it still allowed? Should it be stopped?

It is infant circumcision, a practice instituted four thousand years ago in the Bible. Today thousands of new parents face an agonizing decision; should they or shouldn't they?

The RECAP Solution

R. Wayne Griffiths started a support group called RECAP for men who have been "mutilated" in this way. "There are a lot of men," he said, "who are enraged that they were violated without their consent and they want to do something about it."[6] Mr. Griffiths decided to take action. He invented a seven-and-one-half-ounce skin-stretcher that "looks like a tiny steel barbell," and he hung this from his "amputation site" for "four to twelve hours every day, except weekends." After eighteen months he had reached his goal. "I'm fully covered and have some overhang," he declared.[7]

Tongue-in-cheek, I (DES) decided to do a little survey of my patients:[8]

"Are you enraged about being circumcised?" I asked.

"What?" they said.

When I explained about RECAP, they looked at me as if I was from the dark side of the moon. I'm sure these enraged men exist but I just couldn't find any who had even thought about this issue.

Light or Heat

In the early 1900s, Americans generally accepted biblical traditions, so the practice of circumcision flourished. As the century progressed, however, many physicians developed hostility toward biblical traditions. Some supercharged the issue by asking parents, "Would you prefer to leave your son *intact* or have his *foreskin amputated?*"

Our procircumcision writings also ignited emotional responses. People wrote us ten-page letters and scolded us in full-length books. One author wrote that she was "surprised to see this approach from Christians."

With the fiery debates raging, many parents have agonized over their own decisions. Rather than add kindling to the fire, maybe in all this heat we can find some light.

Why would anyone inflict "genital mutilation" on a little baby? During the 1960s many doctors wondered that themselves. This seemingly unnecessary suffering spurred the American Academy of Pediatrics to issue an emphatic statement in 1971: "There are no valid medical indications for circumcision in the neonatal period."[9]

Soon anticircumcision became a New Age religious doctrine. The baby was a "helpless victim"! Some crusaded for these abused boys as if they were whales, seals, or spotted owls.

Doctors pleaded, "Stop the 'Rape of the Phallus,'"[10] and, "Put an end to the 'Penile Plunder.'"[11] Hearing these slogans, many parents decided not to "mutilate" their sons.

In the early 1980s most of my (DES) medical professors laughed when I suggested the issue might have another side. Did I also want to go back to bloodletting and leeches?

Dr. Semmelweis Lives Again

About this time, an energetic pediatrician, Dr. Thomas Wiswell, joined the anticircumcision crusade: "Circumcision was a dirty word. I became an outspoken opponent of the procedure. I felt, as did many pediatricians, analogous to . . . a knight warding off the evil dragon circumcision."[12]

Dr. Wiswell specialized in newborn intensive care. Here he spent thousands of hours caring for frail, sick newborns. As Dr. Semmelweis had, Wiswell began looking for ways to prevent deadly infections.

One day while reviewing the hospital records of 200,000 newborn boys, he noticed a startling trend. Uncircumcised boys were ten times more likely than circumcised boys to suffer urinary tract infections.[13] Doctors had been crusading against circumcision but they had overlooked the lethal results. As the number of uncircumcised infants doubled, the rate of serious urinary tract infections had also doubled.

Many dismissed Dr. Wiswell's findings, because (as one doctor said) they had "no plausible explanation."[14]

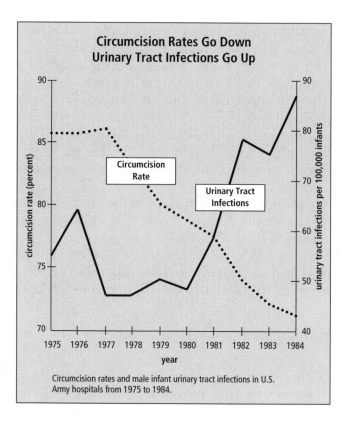

**Circumcision Rates Go Down
Urinary Tract Infections Go Up**

Circumcision rates and male infant urinary tract infections in U.S. Army hospitals from 1975 to 1984.

Dr. Wiswell published a complete review of circumcision complications.[15] Still one critic said, "Wiswell (with a name made for himself and a position to defend?) . . . refuses to admit that any complications of circumcision exist."[16]

He did the most thorough research ever on the subject, yet listen to one detractor: "Wiswell summarily dismisses any refutations of his findings without any fair or objective consideration of the matter."[17] One would hardly recognize this Dr. Wiswell as the doctor who, after publishing his original study, cautioned, "As of this time, we do not recommend routine circumcision of the newborn."[18]

Unlike Semmelweis, Wiswell was not fired and he continued to do research on the issue. Over the next few years, nine different studies found circumcision to protect against urinary tract infections. Indeed circumcision may be the best way to prevent these infections.

Africa and the Plague

While Dr. Wiswell was making these discoveries, an epidemic of AIDS was spreading across Africa. Millions of Africans became infected, 90 percent of them through heterosexual contact. Up to 80 percent of African prostitutes carried the virus. AIDS orphaned one in ten Ugandan children.

Newsweek captured the tragedy:[19]

Africa in the Plague Years

Several hundred thousand are dead and perhaps 5 million more carry the AIDS virus

Three years ago, 600 Ugandans lived in this settlement not far from the Tanzanian border. They seined Nile perch from Lake Victoria and traded textiles and tea to smugglers from the south. They also traded in sex. The dusty main street . . . was lined with discos full of prostitutes offering "cut-rate sex."

In 1982 AIDS swept through like a prairie fire. Now there are only 150 people left in Kasensero; more than 100 villagers died, and many others left. Today many of the huts are empty.

Funerals are . . . depressingly frequent. . . . Nurse Josephine Naruyima opened up . . . a bamboo dispensary, eight by eight feet. "Since I came here [this year]," she says, "48 people died from 'slim' [AIDS]. . . . We buried a barmaid last week. She was the latest victim, and we hope the last." But seven of the discos are still in business, and the barmaids inside seem to have plenty of customers.

It has become a cliché to call AIDS a plague, but for central Africa no other word is quite as apt.

Why this horrible plague? All the reasons are not yet in, but in 1988 scientists were startled by what they called an "interesting and unexpected" observation.[20] Uncircumcised men were up to eight times more likely to become infected with AIDS.[21]

In Africa AIDS spreads mostly among tribes that do not practice circumcision.[22] You can see this on the map of Africa below. Where circumcision is common, AIDS is rare. Where circumcision is rare, AIDS is common.

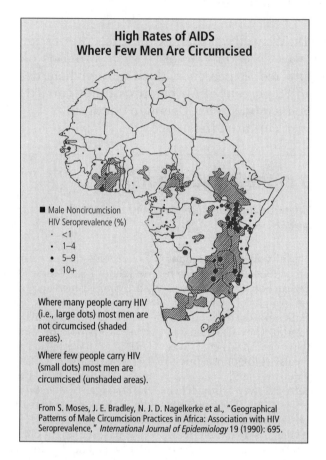

**High Rates of AIDS
Where Few Men Are Circumcised**

■ Male Noncircumcision
HIV Seroprevalence (%)
· <1
· 1–4
● 5–9
● 10+

Where many people carry HIV (i.e., large dots) most men are not circumcised (shaded areas).

Where few people carry HIV (small dots) most men are circumcised (unshaded areas).

From S. Moses, J. E. Bradley, N. J. D. Nagelkerke et al., "Geographical Patterns of Male Circumcision Practices in Africa: Association with HIV Seroprevalence," *International Journal of Epidemiology* 19 (1990): 695.

But this finding should have surprised no one. Almost fifty studies have found the moist, thin foreskin much more susceptible to all kinds of sexually transmitted diseases.[23] Thomas Quinn of the National Institutes of Health comments, "The finding suggests that circumcision should be advocated, just as we advocate condoms. We've got to do everything we can to decrease . . . [AIDS] transmission."[24]

Of course, circumcision and condoms are not the best protection against AIDS. God's command to keep sex within marriage protects against AIDS for sure (see chapter 15). But Africa proves that if every male is circumcised, a population has fairly good (though far from perfect) protection against AIDS.

Vaccinations use this same concept of partial protection. If everyone is partially protected, many epidemics can be kept in check. Thus circumcision can be seen as a way to "vaccinate" a society against AIDS. This dramatically reduces the number of AIDS carriers and, thus, the number of innocent victims within a population.

The Question of Cancer

The protective effects of circumcision have been long known. As far back as 1932 Dr. A. L. Wolburst found that circumcision protects against the often fatal penile cancer. He reviewed hundreds of cases and made a startling discovery. Of 1,103 cancers, not a single case occurred in a Jewish man.

Why were Jews protected? Almost four thousand years ago God told Abraham to circumcise every male child. Since then, Jews have faithfully circumcised every generation. Dr. Wolburst suspected that this circumcision protected Jewish men against penile cancer.

Since then three large studies have proven Dr. Wolburst's hunch. In over 521 men with penile cancer, not a single circumcised man was found.[25] Worldwide since 1930, doctors have not reported even ten circumcised men with penile cancer. Penile cancer stands alone as the only cancer that can be virtually eliminated by a simple preventive procedure—circumcision. It is 99.9 percent effective in preventing this horrible disease.

That's tremendous! After years of research, science has demonstrated the most effective way to prevent infant urinary tract infections and penile cancer. But science did not arrive at this conclusion because of any laboratory steam it had generated. No! A long train of statistics pulled science up discovery hill. These statistics existed only because generations had followed God's command to circumcise every infant boy.

Organized Medicine Does a Double Take

It took some time, but even the American Academy of Pediatrics started to come around. Remember their statement of 1971: "There are no valid medical indications for circumcision in the neonatal period."[26] By 1989 their statement had changed:

> Properly performed newborn circumcision prevents [penile problems] . . . and has been shown to decrease the incidence of [penile] cancer. . . . It may result in a decreased incidence of urinary tract infections. . . . Newborn circumcision is a rapid and generally safe procedure when performed by an experienced operator. . . .
>
> Newborn circumcision has potential medical benefits and advantages as well as disadvantages and risks. When circumcision is being considered, the benefits and risks should be explained to the parents and informed consent obtained.[27]

What an amazing turn around! In less than two decades, they reversed their stand. They no longer say, "No valid indication." Now they list the benefits and recommend that parents give "informed consent," as required for all medical procedures.

1971	1989
"There are no valid medical indications for circumcision in the neonatal period."	"Newborn circumcision has potential medical benefits and advantages. . . ."
The American Academy of Pediatrics	*The American Academy of Pediatrics*

Dr. Edgar Schoen, the original chairman of the Task Force on Circumcision, has completely changed his mind: "Largely on the basis of subsequent publications, I personally agree with

Dr. Wiswell that current evidence indicates that the *benefits of newborn circumcision outweigh the risks* of the procedure."[28] What an amazing statement! Remember, this man's original Task Force had concluded that newborn circumcision had "no valid medical indications."

Things moved so much faster than they did in the days of Dr. Semmelweis. Dr. Wiswell has lived to see his conclusions vindicated.

"Religion, Not Science"

Nonetheless, some retreat to attacking circumcision because it is a "ritualistic" and "cruel" practice, "rooted in traditional and cultural values":

> Obviously, circumcision originates from religion, not from science. Would any institutional ethics committee have approved experimental surgical removal of the foreskin of male infants in an attempt to decrease urinary tract infections or even cancer?[29]

Indeed! Doctors would never have thought of setting up an experiment to research the benefits of cutting off foreskins. Rather, the "experiment" was designed in God's ancient health manual, the Bible.

As the third millennium approached, science finally closed in on the experiment's results: "none of these diseases."

Note: If you are an expectant parent, please refer to the appendix for some guidelines in making your own personal decision for your baby boy.

NINE

The Mystery of the Eighth Day

Today the world is at the threshold of what progressive young adults are calling the New Age. . . . The non-circumcision movement is but one outward symbol of a tremendous upheaval presently taking place in human consciousness . . . this all encompassing process of spiritual enlightenment. . . .

Jeffrey R. Wood
(c. 1990)

For generations every male among you who is eight days old must be circumcised. . . . My covenant in your flesh is to be an everlasting covenant.

God, Gen. 17:12–13
(c. 1900 B.C.)

While I (SIM) was practicing medicine in West Africa, the chief of a local tribe awakened me in the middle of the night. I could hardly believe my ears; he wanted me to get up immediately and circumcise his twelve-year-old son. In Africa you do not argue with the chief, so I performed the late-night circumcision. He warned me to keep the surgery secret.

Two weeks later another midnight messenger awakened me and told me to follow him. Silently the two of us stole down a narrow jungle path. As we neared a clearing, the drums banged out a haunting beat. For several hours the boys danced around a large bonfire. In the eerie shadows, their painted chests and faces reflected the flickering light.

Then the drums stopped. The boys trembled as they lined up. A large butcher knife in hand, the witch doctor approached. Inside a wild lion-faced mask, he roared ferociously as he paced up and down the line. Suddenly he stopped at the first boy, ripped off the boy's loincloth, grasped his foreskin, shrieked a hideous cry, jumped into the air, and sliced off his foreskin. Shaking with terror, each boy screamed as his turn came. Then he doubled over and moaned in pain.

Last in line was the chief's son. He walked off with the witch doctor. The two of them entered a small hut. We heard the witch doctor's loud shriek but no cry of pain from the boy. While the rest were still writhing in pain, the chief's son walked out nonchalantly. He jumped on a donkey and rode into the village.

No one realized that he had been circumcised almost two weeks before. Marveling at his mettle, everyone agreed that this boy was going to make a great chief.

The Pain Factor

As those boys could testify, circumcision hurts. Because of this pain, maybe parents should wait until boys can make the decision for themselves.

According to "The Infant's and Young Child's Bill of Rights":

> A little boy has the right not only to keep his foreskin but to have it left entirely alone. . . . Such procedures should be reserved for older individuals (teenagers and adults) who are able to make such personal decisions for themselves.[1]

But is waiting really humane? Even when circumcised in a modern hospital, twelve year olds suffer pain for about a week. Newborns, on the other hand, are extremely resilient. Within minutes they finish crying and are ready to feed. By the age of three months, however, circumcision causes pain and irritability for three or four days.[2]

In addition to pain, imagine the emotional trauma for a preteen who has just begun discovering his own sexuality. Think of his confusion and anger at this apparent assault on his sex organs. Unless a medical problem needs correction, no boy should be circumcised after infancy. If you don't do it then, you shouldn't do it later.

Unfortunately, up to 10 percent of boys left uncircumcised will develop a medical problem and will need circumcision later in life. It hurts just to think about it.

The most humane time to circumcise is in the first month of life. After that it is just too painful. It's not a matter of rights. It is simply a matter of compassion.

Infection Insurance

In the United States, circumcisions currently prevent more than ten thousand infant urinary tract infections (UTI) per year. If these boys were not circumcised, these infections would kill up to two hundred boys.[3] When God gave the ancient command to circumcise, no one knew about antibiotics, so these infections were much more serious. Ten thousand infections would have resulted in over two thousand deaths. Infant circumcision saves lives today, but in the days of Abraham it saved many more.

Of course if we wait for the boys to make their own decisions, some will simply die as infants, never having the opportunity to make a decision. The so-called right to decide for himself sounds pretty hollow to the mother of a baby who has just died of a urinary tract infection.

Day Eight, Not a Moment Too Late

When western physicians began circumcising babies, they did it during the first few days of life while the baby was still in the hospital. Occasionally one would bleed severely. Rarely a boy would bleed to death. For a long time, physicians were puzzled by this serious bleeding. What was going on?

Finally, in the early 1900s scientists began to solve the chemistry of blood clotting and they found the answer. The body needs vitamin K to make clotting proteins. Newborn babies, however, don't start making vitamin K until they are five days old. As a result, by a baby's third day one clotting protein (prothrombin) drops to 30 percent of normal. In a pediatric journal we read, "The greatest risk [of bleeding] occurs between two and seven days of life."[4] According to a textbook, bleeding at this time "may produce serious damage to internal organs, especially to the brain, and cause death from shock and exsanguination."[5]

Soon after birth, the baby begins to produce vitamin K.[6] By day eight, prothrombin levels jump back to 110 percent of the adult level. Thus the safest day for circumcision in a baby's life is day eight.[7]

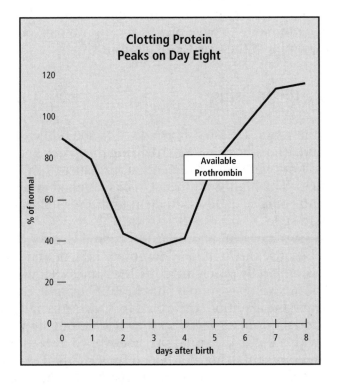

As we marvel at the wonders of modern science, we can almost hear the pages of our Bibles rustling to Genesis 17:12 where God says to Abraham, "Every boy must be circumcised on the eighth day. . . ."

Who picked the eighth day, the most humane and safest moment in a boy's life? Modern medical textbooks sometimes suggest that the Hebrews conducted careful observations of bleeding tendencies.[8] Yet what is the evidence? Severe bleeding occurs at most in only 1 out of 200 babies.[9] Determining the safest day for circumcision would have required careful experiments, observing thousands of circumcisions. Could Abraham (a primitive, desert-dwelling nomad) have done that?

Maybe a more reasonable explanation for eighth day circumcision is the Bible's statement, "God spoke to Abraham." Historians believe that infant circumcision was unique to the Israelites. Thus neither Abraham, his family, nor any of his neighbors had undergone infant circumcision. Who do you think is more likely to have picked the eighth day: an ancient medical genius or the Creator of vitamin K?

Revising the Incising

Over the years, Jewish rabbis added to the biblical circumcision ritual (i.e., the *Brit Milah*). During the Greek and Roman Empires, Jews were under tremendous pressure to give up their Jewishness. The highly cultured Greeks laughed at the "backward" and "barbaric" Jews. Racism and anti-Semitism were actually in style.

Some Jews caved in and tried to become Greeks. This was difficult because the minute a Jew entered the public baths his circumcision loudly proclaimed his Jewishness. How could he hide? The answer was simple but painful; burn the remaining foreskin and the resulting scar would form an artificial foreskin.

This horrified many Jews, so they decided to stop it. After cutting with a knife, the ritual surgeon ripped away any of the remaining foreskin using sharpened fingernails. This assured a permanent, heavily scarred circumcision site. Unfortunately, this ritual (the *Priah*) left a ragged wound, delaying healing and risking infection.

By the seventh century A.D., ritual surgeons had added the *metzitza* or sucking out. Here the operator moistened his lips with wine and sucked blood out of the ragged wound. Some say they did this "for the purpose of cleansing the area and removing germs which might harm the infant."[10] They considered infants to be in "mortal danger" if the sucking out was not performed. Even the great Jewish physician Maimonides endorsed the *metzitza* to prevent infection.[11]

Today we know that the sucking out did not protect anyone. Instead, it exposed the fragile infant to a slew of dangerous mouth germs. From a medical viewpoint, it effectively turned a clean surgery into an infection-prone human bite. Even today, ritual surgeons are infecting babies with fatal cases of gangrene, tuberculosis, and tetanus.[12] The specter of AIDS has created the frightening possibility of a ritual surgeon infecting hundreds of babies with the AIDS virus.[13]

But what did the ritual look like originally? God commanded them to use a *new "flint knife"* (Josh. 5:2). They made a flint knife by chipping away stone fragments, producing a clean, sharp edge. The exposed rock is germ-free. Instead of this clean and safe technique, the later additions of scraping and sucking out turned it into a dirty and dangerous ritual.

Isn't it interesting that Moses didn't recommend an Egyptian manure ointment, to "speed up the healing"? Moses simply stuck to the divine directions. God's way was the best way. God's method helped healing, limited bleeding, and prevented infection.

That's the mystery of the eighth day: "none of these diseases . . ."

SEXUAL WHOLENESS

TEN

Born Gay?

"Derrick Davis—HIV: Positive (confirmed by Western Blot)." I (DES) see a similar lab report all too often; every time it seems so tragic. I phoned Derrick, a local restaurant owner, to come in and discuss his tests.

Derrick rushed right in. He was wringing his hands and dripping with sweat. "Don't tell me, Doc. I know. I've got it; don't I?"

"That's what the test says," I replied.

"Can we repeat it?" he asked.

"Sure," I said.

Tears ran down his cheeks as he recounted his story.

At the age of eleven, he spent the summer with his eighteen-year-old cousin, Gary. Sharing his room, Gary introduced him to the thrills and chills of sexual play. The episodes left him ashamed, excited, and angry—but mainly confused.

Later, as a teenager, he dated only girls. He met his wife Jane in college. During the first few years of marriage, there were some rocky times, but it was "mostly a good marriage." Then one evening after working late, two waitresses invited Derrick out for a drink. They were open lesbians and they took him to a gay bar. Derrick's presence set off an instant sexual feeding frenzy among the bar regulars. Within thirty minutes, three men had asked him out. The attention was intoxicating.

He spent three hours with one man, discussing music, food, and sex. After several drinks, Derrick left the bar with Larry. The morning after, Derrick awoke in a strange bed with a strange man lovingly stroking his hair.

Again those confusing feelings surfaced. He was ashamed, yet "it seemed so loving." He didn't understand his anger. "It was," he said, "the most tender anger I ever felt."

Despite his confusion, Derrick often returned to Larry's bed. Homosexual thoughts dominated his time. On many a night he found anonymous sex through a hole in a bathroom stall.

His feelings toward Jane changed. Almost everything she did bothered him. She wanted time. She wanted romance. She wanted intimacy. But he wanted out. The idea of having sex with any woman became repulsive.

Finally, he announced that he was "gay," and the marriage was over. "I don't want to hurt you," he told her, "but I can't change. It's who I really am. . . . I can't live a lie anymore."

Then he walked out on Jane, his four-year-old son, and his infant daughter. He traded the safety and fulfillment of marriage for the risk and emptiness of a thousand nameless partners.

In my office he realized that his choice would also end his life. "Why me?" he wept. "I was always so careful. I always used a condom."

That night he told Larry about the blood test, and Larry walked right out the door. The fleeting thrill of a bathroom stall had flushed Derrick's life down the drain. Following another script, he could have still enjoyed kissing his children good night and sleeping soundly in bed with his wife. Instead, for a hundred sleepless nights he tossed and wondered who had given him the kiss of death.

He felt the despair of King Solomon, who after having more than a thousand women, cried out, "Meaningless! Meaningless! . . . Everything is meaningless" (Eccles. 1:1 NIV)

Why John Likes Jack

Derrick's story illustrates the complex nature of sexual orientation. As with Derrick, no one wakes up one morning and suddenly decides, *Today I am going to be gay.* Sexuality is much more subtle and complex. Some, including Ann Landers, hold the trendy opinion that "Human sexual orientation is determined at birth."[1] This popular view, however, has little basis in fact. Research shows that human sexuality is complex but it *definitely is* not *predetermined at birth.*

We don't have all the answers, but at least five factors seem to favor development of homosexual orientation.[2]

Genetics

Genetics may influence homosexual tendencies. There is indeed a growing body of evidence that genes do play some role in sexual orientation. The most important studies are those of identical twins, who share identical genes, but they also have:

- identical parents who treat them very similarly
- identical surroundings
- shared identities

Despite all these similarities in upbringing and a perfect genetic match, if one twin chooses a gay lifestyle, the other twin has *only a 50 percent chance of living gay.* You don't need a degree in genetics to realize that this proves there is no simple "gay gene." Genes may fix eye color, hair color, and skin color, but they do not fix sexual preference. Genes may produce leanings toward homosexuality, but *genes do not cause homosexuality.*

Still, activists try to justify themselves with scientific research. Gay activists rapidly followed one "gay gene" study with a press release, declaring that it proved "Homosexuality is a naturally occurring and common variation among humans."[3] So what! So is depression. So is alcoholism. So is schizophrenia. Even if a condition is "naturally occurring and common," does that make it desirable?

As Charles Krauthammer wrote in the *Washington Post:*

> Science has nothing to say to either side of the gay rights debate. The tolerance or discouragement of homosexuality is a question to be decided according to what people believe about the value, the morality, and the chances for happiness of a homosexual life. The science is irrelevant.[4]

Confusing Sexual Experiences

Confusing sexual experiences may influence homosexual tendencies. Most lesbians, when they were children, were sexually abused by men. These traumatic memories foster a fear of intimacy with men. For boys, early homosexual encounters may cause sexual confusion. Even so, almost all of these boys go on to develop normal heterosexual drives.

During puberty, some children sense vague same-sex attractions. Superficial and fleeting, these twinges usually fade as soon as the child begins to notice the opposite sex. When a school counselor hears of these same-sex twinges, however, he may answer, "That's normal. You must be gay." Now the child is really confused.

I (DES) have met several young men who have received such counsel and then entered gay life, only later to discover the truth. These twinges don't make a boy gay, any more than wagging its tail makes a cat a dog.

Breakdown of the Social Fabric

Breakdown of the social fabric may influence homosexual tendencies. Gay propaganda says that gays are not in the business of recruiting our children. "Either you're gay or you're not," they say. "A leopard can't change his spots." If you have any question whether the gay population is in the business of marketing and selling their lifestyle, let me (DES) recount a Friday night stroll I took in Philadelphia when I was in medical school.

Spruce Street bustled with a sense of excitement. There were the smells of ethnic food and a sporadic whiff of marijuana. Whistles, laughs, and cheers interrupted a guitarist singing strains of Bob Dylan.

I walked by a pay phone. It rang. I naively answered it. "Hello?"

"Hello, friend," a man answered dreamily.

"Who is this?" I asked.

"Someone who wants to have some fun."

"Who are you?" I asked.

"Look up—in the window across the street."

There stood a thin, middle-aged man making sexually suggestive gestures. "Sorry," I said. "I'm straight."

"So what?" he said. "So was I. Had a wife and kids. BOR-RRRING! You don't know what you're missin'. Come on up. We'll have laaawts of fun."

"No thanks," I said.

As I hung up the phone, he sneered, "HET!"[5]

Lonely or insecure young people are easy prey for these homosexual hunters who bait their tragic traps with the promise of instant sexual oohs and aahs. The sexual jungle has never been so dangerous.

When tempted, some otherwise heterosexual men try out homosexual sex. Among prison inmates, about 30 percent practice homosexuality of their own free will. Immediately on release from prison, however, almost all of them return to exclusive heterosexuality. For these men, homosexual intercourse is merely an optional way for sexual release. This illustrates that *homosexuality* describes what someone *does,* not what someone *is.*

Like sewage from a manhole, homosexuality has overflowed into the streets of America. Many young people are trying out the so-called gay life only because our society has allowed the Spruce Streets to exist. We should never have let it happen.

A Distant Father

For both boys and girls, fathers are the most important factor in sexual orientation.[6] More than 80 percent of gay men (but only 18 percent of straight men) have emotionally distant fathers.[7]

Boys who never experienced a dad's masculine hug or back-slap feel a strange mix of love and hatred for their father. They may search for male intimacy elsewhere, but it never satisfies. Ambivalent desires *both to love and to punish* their father set the stage for unstable male relationships.

Unfortunately, many fathers think that being a distant, macho dad will ensure a masculine, heterosexual son. Nothing could be farther from the truth. It actually tends to drive a boy toward homosexuality. Boys with warm relationships with masculine fathers rarely turn to homosexuality. A loving father-son relationship is like a vaccine, immunizing a boy against homosexual orientation.[8]

Every minute a father spends with his sons makes a difference in their lives. Time invested in these boys will help ensure normal moral, intellectual, emotional, and sexual development. That's the kind of relationship that the Bible encourages. Listen to a biblical sage speak of his father: "When I was a boy in my father's house, still tender, and an only child of my mother, he taught me and said, 'Lay hold of my words with all your heart; keep my commands and you will live'" (Prov. 4:3–4 NIV).[9] That's exactly the kind of father relationship every son wants and needs. The Bible directs, "Fathers, don't provoke your children to anger. Instead, nurture them in the discipline and instruction of the Lord" (Eph. 6:4). Fathering like that protects a son against sexual deviation.

A Smothering Mother

A smothering mother who is also a spiteful wife may influence homosexual tendencies. Children destined for the "gay life" tend to have smothering mothers. These mothers often baby and restrict their boys by discouraging sports, preventing dates, and forcing them into girlish activities—such as knitting, sewing, and bubble baths. These boys may still sleep in their mother's bed as teenagers. Many harbor a hidden rage toward their mother for this forced "sissification."

Despite the popular idea that boys and girls are equivalent and interchangeable, study after study has shown that maleness and femaleness are an inborn part of who we are. We are not sort of male or sort of female. Through and through we are either male or female. It takes tremendous pressure to alter our inborn sexual identity.

God made us that way and he intends us to parent that way. Often Baby Boomer parents describe their failures at unisex parenting. One parent noted that she gave her toddler boy a doll, only to find him playing baseball with the head. Boys resist feminization. Girls resist masculinization. Unisex parenting, although a fad, ignores centuries of human wisdom, goes against biblical teaching, and confuses children.

Smothering mothers also tend to be spiteful wives, openly despising and degrading their husbands. They often encourage their sons to take sides against their father. These mothers are nothing like the biblical wife. "She brings [her husband] good, not harm, all the days of her life. . . . Her children arise and call her blessed; her husband also, and he praises her" (Prov. 31:12, 28 NIV). She is no smothering mother. She is no spiteful wife.

When it comes to sex, three out of four mothers of gay men talked about sex as dirty and disgusting—an act serving merely to gratify male animal lust.[10] These moms often justify their frigidity with religious language. This is the reason many psychiatrists blame religion for teaching women to put sex in the deep freeze. What a surprise would await these psychiatrists if they were to read the frank sexual language of the Bible:

> How beautiful you are and how pleasing,
> O love, with your delights!
> Your stature is like that of the palm,
> and your breasts like clusters of fruit.
> I said, "I will climb the palm tree;
> I will take hold of its fruit."
> May your breasts be like the clusters of the vine,
> the fragrance of your breath like apples,
> and your mouth like the best wine.
>
> Song of Songs 7:6–9 NIV

That's almost as explicit as a Madonna video, but it's the Bible. Biblical sexuality is not sexual frigidity but marital fidelity. Biblical sex is as passionate as, but far more meaningful than, any one-night stand. The Bible doesn't store sex in the prude's frigid freezer. Neither does the Bible ignite sex in the gay's blazing bonfire. The Bible lays sex by the glowing fireplace of marriage.

For centuries Jews have used the Song of Songs to openly introduce their teenagers to the wonders of marriage and sexuality. A British scholar notes:

> I had always been struck by the unembarrassed plainness of speech with which they [the Hebrews] discussed sexual matters. But I had not fully realized that it had its roots in an essentially "clean" conception of the essential goodness of the sexual function. This is something very difficult for us to grasp, reared as we have been in a tradition which has produced in many minds the rooted idea that sex is essentially sinful.[11]

Even today Orthodox Jews continue to apply these sexual principles, so it is little wonder that they have low rates of sexual confusion. One researcher noted, "The [frequency of the] homosexual among Orthodox Jewish groups appears to be phenomenally low."[12]

Studies have consistently shown that the *best protection* against future generations of homosexuality is *a family functioning according to biblical principles.* God continues to protect families and societies from the ravages of homosexual behavior, if they "give careful attention to the voice of the Lord. . . . do what is right in his sight, give ear to his commands, and keep all his statutes . . ." (Exod. 15:26).

ELEVEN

Sexual Musical Chairs

Bernard: Yeah, freedom, baby! Freedom!

Larry: You gotta have it! It can't work any other way. And the ones who swear their undying fidelity are lying. Most of them, anyway—ninety percent of them. They cheat on each other constantly and lie through their teeth. I'm sorry, I can't be like that and it drives Hank up the wall.

> Mart Crowley,
> *The Boys in the Band*

Gay activists like to portray themselves as mature, monogamous people who maintain lasting, loving relationships. A few may—but very few. Here are the sad facts. *A full 75 percent of gay men do most of their sex acts with men they don't even know.* About 30 percent of gay men rack up *more than one thousand lifetime partners.*[1]

One man describes his life:

> I wouldn't wish it on my worst enemy. . . . Over the years I lived with a succession of roommates some of whom I professed love. They swore they loved me. But homosexual ties begin and end with sex. There is so little else to go on. After that first passionate fling,

sex becomes less and less frequent. The partners become nervous. They want new thrills, new experiences. They begin to cheat on each other—secretly at first, then more obviously. . . . There are jealous rages and fights. Eventually you split and begin hustling around for a new lover.[2]

The romantic recruit looking for lasting love will find bitter disappointment in a homosexual relationship. Gay love is not love at all. Gay relationships always deteriorate into insecurity, infighting, and infidelity.

Let's look at one study of one hundred "stable" gay couples.[3] After living together for a full five years, not one couple had remained sexually faithful. The authors, a gay couple themselves, conclude that *to be gay is to need multiple partners*. They insist that *lasting, faithful relationships do not exist in the "normal" homosexual lifestyle.*

In essence these researchers say to a man attempting a long-term gay relationship, "Forget it! You are refusing to accept your own homosexuality. Get over your homophobia. When you finally accept your homosexuality, you will spend your life playing nonstop sexual musical chairs."

Humans are different from studs on horse farms and roosters in hen houses. God never intended people to live like animals. Compulsive copulation with countless partners is not normal for human beings. It is a sign of neurosis.

Draw Lines and Build Bridges

The homosexual lifestyle can never be an acceptable alternative to God's creation model. God made humanity "in the image of God . . . male and female" (Gen. 1:27 NIV). Sex is healthy only in the context of God's plan—a marriage between a man and a woman: "A man will leave his father and mother and be united to his wife, and they will become one flesh" (Gen. 2:24 NIV).

God's plan is always the best plan. Even today, only 4 percent of married people commit adultery in a given year.[4] What a contrast with gay couples—100 percent unfaithful in five years!

Religious groups that release statements condoning "faithful homosexual relationships" sound enlightened and compassionate but they describe a virtual reality. Churches might as well release statements condoning the relationship of "Beauty and the Beast." Why condone relationships that do not exist?

The whole idea of the "gay marriage" is fundamentally flawed. Gay men do *not* maintain stable monogamous relationships. The gay marriage movement is not about reality. It is about social acceptance and political power.

It is time to say lovingly but firmly to the egg-throwing activists: "You matter to God and you matter to us, but your ideas for redefining the family are wrong. They are confusing our young people and they are sowing seeds of disease and despair. We have no obligation to endorse your behavior— behavior labeled by Chief Supreme Court Justice Warren Burger as contrary to 'millennia of moral teaching.'[5] In fact we have every obligation to condemn such behavior. We don't hate you. But your behavior is not gay; it's sad. It's not beneficial; it's destructive. It's not right; it's wrong."

God calls people of faith to draw lines and build bridges[6]— to set boundaries and reach out to those living outside those boundaries. We do not condone the wrong by caring for the wrongdoer. Physicians do not condone murder by sewing up a murderer's wounds. We do not condone homosexual acts by reaching out in compassion to a person with AIDS.

If Jesus were walking the earth today, we might find him in an AIDS ward. While he walked the earth, he always seemed to show up where sinners were suffering. He often hung around prostitutes and so-called lowlifes. He never kicked people when they were down; he lifted them up. He didn't seem so worried about how they got there; he was more concerned about where they were going. We believe Jesus is calling his followers to do the same today.

Sex has boundaries. God's love has no boundaries. His love always extends even to those who have strayed far across sexual boundaries.

The Homosexual Neurosis

Why do some choose to live outside sexual boundaries? Why do they seek out hundreds of same-sex partners? Could it be evidence of a psychological problem?

Since the beginning of psychiatry, doctors held that homosexuality was a disorder. But in 1974 the American Psychiatric Association caved in to the activists who constantly disrupted their meetings. They got the activists off their backs by declaring that homosexuality was no longer a psychological disturbance. But giving in to political protests rarely makes for good science. Since then, researchers have found boatloads of data, showing that homosexuals definitely swim outside the psychological mainstream. Whatever the test, wherever the country, and whomever the social group—researchers have consistently found the same result. Homosexual men score abnormally high on tests measuring for neurosis.[7]

Practicing homosexuals tend to display the following neurotic traits:

- *A sense of inferiority:* An inferiority complex comes naturally to a boy who never received his dad's approval and whose mother constantly pushed him into feminine activities, making him feel inferior to other boys. Thus other boys seemed much more masculine or attractive. Feeling inferior, he begins to admire other boys. This *adoration of other boys* later grows into same-sex desires.
- *Self-centeredness:* Homosexual "love" is nothing like the joyful experience of falling in love. Rather, it is a neurotic compulsion to drain love out of the lover. Self-centered or narcissistic, it strives *to get love not to give love.*
- *Sexual obsession:* Homosexual thoughts dominate the gay man's thought life, much like the drug addict's drug-oriented thought life.
- *Self-pity:* One thought constantly torments the homosexual: "It's not fair." He is likely to worry or whine about his physical appearance, some "nervous crisis," a health worry,

or society's "homophobia." This constant complaining explains why the gay minority, less than 3 percent of the population, produces such vocal political protest.

- *Compulsive craving:* Same-sex "love" is never satisfied. It is much like the kleptomaniac who constantly shoplifts—not because he needs more things, but because he has an obsessive compulsion to steal. That is why a gay man gets caught in a whirlwind of sexual exploits—not because he needs more partners, but because he has an obsessive compulsion for sex.

- *Anger:* The gay man is torn between desire for the dad he never had and anger at the father he really had. Lying with his partner, he longs for a close male relationship. Fighting with his partner, he rages at an absent father.

A New Diagnosis

In the past decade psychologists have introduced the idea of "sexual addiction." Of course it is simplistic to equate cocaine craving with neurotic lust, yet the model may be useful in developing programs to help these "sex addicts."

In an article in *Postgraduate Medicine,* Dr. Jennifer Schneider lists the three hallmarks of the sex addict:

- *Compulsion:* One feels unable to stop his reckless sex life.
- *Persistence:* One continues reckless sex despite negative effects on his life, such as sexually transmitted diseases or divorce.
- *Obsession:* One feels unable to curb a constant sexual preoccupation.[8]

Sound familiar?

Today the politically correct term is *sexual addiction.* Of course, *the homosexual neurosis is a sexual addiction.* Psychiatrists no longer label homosexuality a disorder. But in today's politically correct world one can simply label homosexuality as *"same-sex sexual addiction."* No matter what you call it, the homosexual lifestyle remains unnatural, unhealthy, and psychologically abnormal.

One man suffering from AIDS summarized his feelings, "I'm already living under my own judgment, I don't need you to judge me." Indeed, homosexuals don't need hate; they need help. Many may not want help, but hate only breeds more hate.

They have popularized the idea that theirs is a gay (as in happy) lifestyle. But after hearing the stories of practicing gays over the years, we have seen the truth. Their lives are empty and unfulfilling. As a character in the play *The Boys in the Band* says, "You show me a happy homosexual, and I'll show you a gay corpse."[9]

Randy's Prom

Randy Rohl didn't want that kind of life for himself. His life had been difficult with his parents splitting up when he was only six. His mom said, "I knew Randy was different but I didn't know why." He always wanted to get a reaction out of people. In hallways he might bark, and then look at you and say, "Knock it off."

In 1979 he got a reaction out of the entire country when he and Grady Quinn became the first same-sex couple to attend an American high school prom. With TV camera lights glaring, the couple danced the night away in matching powder blue tuxedos, red rose boutonnieres, and silver pierced earrings. TV and newspapers proclaimed that the American prom was finally "out of the closet."

But things have changed. In 1994 it wasn't even big news when the Los Angeles School District actually sponsored an all-gay prom. Same-sex boy, girl, and drag queen couples arrived in limos at the Los Angeles Hilton, where the *L.A. Times* reported that they "smooched, dined, and danced this close."[10] Parents of one gay teen gushed about the event, "The ballroom was beautifully decorated, the chaperones supportive, and the young faces radiant with pride. As it should be."[11]

What these parents didn't know was that Randy the "gay pride pioneer" was no longer dancing. On the previous New Year's Eve Randy had missed all the parties. In his home there were no cameras, no reporters, no tuxedos, no boutonnieres, and no glaring lights. Randy wasn't dancing or even smiling. Blind in one eye, he was bedridden. At 10:52 P.M. he died.

On his square that was part of the AIDS memorial quilt, his mother stitched a poem:

> With tearful eyes we watched him linger,
>   and saw him slowly fade away.
> Although we loved him dearly,
>   we could not make him stay.[12]

"A Lesson in Tolerance"

People magazine called a gay prom couple, a "lesson in tolerance." Today many worship at this altar of "tolerance." Talk show hosts act as televangelists for this trendy religion of tolerance, where anything goes.

If anyone dares mention that homosexual practices are wrong or even dangerous, gay activists diagnose him or her as suffering from the social disease of homophobia. They denounce anyone who holds differing moral values as "intolerant." Ironically, these priests of tolerance can't tolerate anyone with different moral values.[13]

What happens if we tolerate what God forbids? The gravestone to the last half of the twentieth century should read:

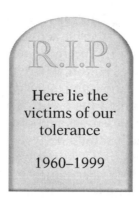

R.I.P.

Here lie the
victims of our
tolerance

1960–1999

Randy's life and the lives of thousands of others are indeed a lesson about tolerance—a lesson that this kind of tolerance produces no social headway, only headlines and headstones.

Is Help Possible?

Despite society's newfound tolerance, about 60 percent of gay men will turn to some form of counseling.[14] Today if a gay man seeks therapy, most therapists will work toward self-acceptance. Even if he says he wants to change, the message will be, "There is nothing wrong with you. You just need to accept and enjoy your sexual preference."

Point	*Counterpoint*
Don't claim . . . that homosexuals can change—we can't and we wouldn't want to if we could. Larry Kramer, gay activist, founder of Act Up, who died of AIDS	The general view in the gay community that treatment is never successful is without foundation. The fact that most homosexual preferences are probably learned and not inborn means that, in the presence of strong motivation to change, they are open to modification, and clinical experience confirms this. Dr. Judd Marmor, psychiatrist

But why? Do we treat any other self-destructive process this way? Do we say to the alcoholic, "That's just who you are. We can treat your hangovers and family problems, but drinking alcohol is part of who you are. Don't try to change. Just accept and enjoy your drinking preference."

Homosexuals, like alcoholics, should not surrender and accept their illness. They need help. They need change. Indeed, therapists have documented many cases of complete reversal of sexual orientation. Harvard psychiatrist Dr. Lee Birk counseled fourteen homosexual men who wished to change their sexual orientation. Ten of these fourteen were so successful that they initiated and maintained "stable and apparently happy marriages."[15]

Rather than see these studies as offering hope, activists prefer to point out failures and relapses, mistaking them for proof that change is impossible. Yet failures and relapses are common to treatment of all neuroses. Should it surprise us that men tend to revert to a long-standing, neurotic sexuality? What if a therapist took the same approach with alcoholics and told them, "Many people relapse, so I can't help you much. Alcoholism is normal. You just have to live with it"? With any disease, modest cure rates don't prove that cures are impossible. They merely show that cures are difficult.

Support groups all over the world offer hope to people suffering all sorts of addictions and neuroses. We should not abandon those caught in the homosexual neurosis. They need to hear the message: Yes, there is help for strugglers of every stripe—including sexual strugglers who desire recovery and wholeness.

The Message of Hope

Still, many feel trapped in the game of sexual musical chairs. In their mind, they hear the blaring music of sexual obsession. Every time it crescendos, they have another nameless encounter. All the while, they live in fear of AIDS. Will the climactic trumpets suddenly stop? On the only chair left, will the Grim Reaper sit?

The message of the Bible is that the human race is a colossal collection of moral failures. All of us fail to live up to our own moral codes. Calling our failures "natural" does not make failure good or unchangeable. Dr. M. Scott Peck has said, "It is also natural to defecate in our pants and never brush our teeth. Yet we teach ourselves to do the unnatural until the unnatural becomes natural."[16] All of life is a struggle against what comes naturally to us.

It was no different in the first century, when Paul described, ". . . sexually immoral . . . sexually unfaithful . . . participants in homosexual acts . . . thieves . . . greedy . . . and alcoholics" (1 Cor. 6:9–10).

But Paul had a message of hope for sexual strugglers: "A number of you know from experience what I'm talking about, for not so long ago you were on that list. Since then, you've been *cleaned up and given a fresh start* by Jesus, our Master, our Messiah, and by our God present in us, the Spirit" (1 Cor. 6:11 *The Message*, italics added).

Since its very beginning, the church has been a gathering of strugglers. Jesus himself said: "Who needs a doctor: the healthy or the sick? I'm here inviting outsiders, not insiders—an invitation to a changed life, changed inside and out" (Luke 5:31–32 *The Message*). Even today many have experienced recovery from homosexual neuroses through a vibrant, healing faith in the power of God.

After treating more than one hundred homosexual men and women, Dr. Gerard van den Aardweg comments, "A religious conversion can afford a homosexual the hope and energy he wants for his struggle."[17]

All of us fight an ongoing struggle against different types of moral failure. To one degree or another, we are all in a state of recovery. Thank God! The power of "God present in us, the Spirit," is available to anyone who wants to be "cleaned up and given a fresh start."

AIDS: Myths or Facts?

Here's a little quiz about the facts of AIDS. The correct answers follow. Give yourself a point for each correct answer.

1. Myth or Fact: The Supreme Court has ruled that the government may not interfere in sexual acts between consenting adults.
2. Myth or Fact: The spread of AIDS in the United States is increasing fastest in rural areas and small cities.
3. Myth or Fact: Women do not really need to worry about AIDS.

4. Myth or Fact: AIDS is easily spread during heterosexual intercourse.
5. Myth or Fact: You are safe if your partner tests negative for HIV.
6. Myth or Fact: Condoms frequently fail to prevent pregnancy and the spread of sexually transmitted diseases (STDs).
7. Myth or Fact: The majority of AIDS cases are transmitted by homosexual acts or illicit drug use.
8. Myth or Fact: God loves people with AIDS.
9. Myth or Fact: Unless one accepts homosexuality as normal, one cannot minister meaningfully to men who acquired AIDS through homosexual acts.
10. Myth or Fact: You are homophobic if you condemn homosexual acts.

AIDS: The Facts

1. Myth. Reality: In 1986 *(Powers v. Hardwick)*, the Supreme Court ruled just the opposite. "The Constitution does not confer a fundamental right upon homosexuals to engage in sodomy."[18]
2. Fact. The growth of the AIDS epidemic is increasing fastest in rural areas and small cities.
3. Myth. Reality: Worldwide, AIDS is split evenly between men and women.
4. Fact. Heterosexual transmission of HIV from men to women and women to men is quite efficient.
5. Myth. Reality: It often takes six months (rarely much longer) after HIV infection for the AIDS test to turn positive.
6. Fact. Many cases of AIDS have been transmitted to and from people who use condoms faithfully.
7. Myth. Reality: Worldwide, about 90 percent of AIDS cases are spread by heterosexual intercourse. The United States is just now beginning to catch up with the rest of the world.

8. Fact. God's love reaches out to any who are suffering, no matter why they are suffering.
9. Myth. Reality. Jesus chose to spend much of his time with the outcast sinners of his day but he never condoned their sinful lifestyles. His followers should do the same.
10. Myth. Reality: This is an ingenious defense: "What's the matter with you? I don't have a problem (homosexual behavior). If you think that I have a problem, *you* must have a problem (homophobia)." But must I have a *phobia* (i.e., an irrational fear) to consider something wrong? If I condemn cigarette smoking, do I have "cigophobia"? There are many reasons (moral convictions, negative consequences, etc.) other than phobias to condemn certain behaviors.

Scoring:

0–5 correct, try AIDgain
6–7 correct, AIDept
8–9 correct, AIDucated
10 correct, AIDSpert

TWELVE

AIDS—Everyone's Problem

Everything is getting worse and worse in AIDS, and all of us have been underestimating it. . . . I don't know of any greater killer than AIDS.

Dr. Halfdan Mahler,
Director of the
World Health Organization

When AIDS first struck, many felt safe. It was a "problem for other people"—homosexuals, heroin addicts, Haitians, and hemophiliacs.

Some pronounced AIDS as God's punishment on homosexuals. They even denounced funding for AIDS research, calling it an outright gift to the gay community. Others put their faith in science. AIDS was merely a momentary blip in the graph of medical progress. The high priests of science would soon work a miracle cure for AIDS. Short of a cure, maybe we could expect a vaccine. In 1986, 74 percent of Americans wishfully expected scientists to develop an AIDS vaccine within ten years.[1]

Even with no vaccine and no miracle cure, most of us felt safe. Scientists and the media encouraged our smugness. *U.S. News and World*

Report (16 May 1986) boldly announced, "Most experts have ... concluded that the virus will not spread widely in the heterosexual population." Most experts were dead wrong.

AIDS and the Heterosexual

Americans stopped hitting the snooze button on the AIDS alarm when Mr. Heterosexual, Magic Johnson, admitted that he could have caught the virus from any one of a hundred women. But even as the epidemic raced into the heterosexual population, some authorities still pretended that it wasn't so. They told the *Washington Post* in 1994, "The disease (AIDS) is unlikely to become widespread in the general population."[2]

Today what they thought *unlikely* is rapidly becoming a *reality*. In the United States, *heterosexual intercourse is the fastest growing way to catch HIV.* Around the world, *over 90 percent of AIDS cases are spread by heterosexual intercourse.*

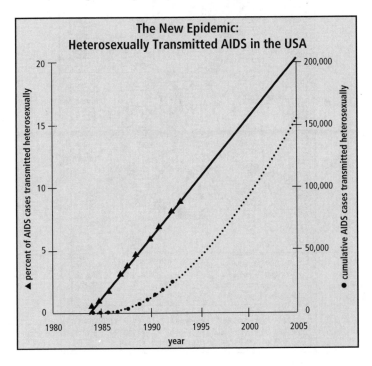

"Gay" sex may be a great way to spread HIV, but straight sex works almost as well. Women have infected millions of men. Men have infected millions of women. You are at risk unless you have had *only one lifetime partner,* who has *never had sex with another person.*

AIDS and Women

Worldwide, AIDS is just as common among women as men. In the United States, AIDS infections are increasing more rapidly among *young women* than any other group.

If you think that this is hype, consider the case of one HIV-positive man and his nineteen women partners. None used

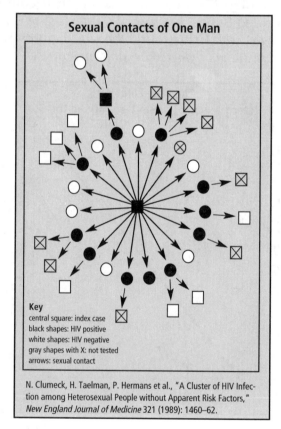

Sexual Contacts of One Man

Key
central square: index case
black shapes: HIV positive
white shapes: HIV negative
gray shapes with X: not tested
arrows: sexual contact

N. Clumeck, H. Taelman, P. Hermans et al., "A Cluster of HIV Infection among Heterosexual People without Apparent Risk Factors," *New England Journal of Medicine* 321 (1989): 1460–62.

drugs. None were prostitutes. None had received a blood transfusion. Only four had subsequently slept with more than one partner. Most were white middle-class, thirty-something women. Almost half were married. They all felt themselves to be at low risk for HIV.

Can you imagine their fear when social workers knocked on their doors and told them that they had been exposed to HIV? Can you imagine the horror of the eleven women when they discovered that they had caught HIV? One woman had already spread it to her partner (see the figure on previous page). Two of these women had only known this man as a one-night stand.

AIDS and Teens

More than a gay disease, today HIV is becoming a teen disease. Every year HIV finds younger and younger victims. *Soon, most HIV may be caught during the teen years.*[3]

MTV warns them. Teachers warn them. Parents warn them. But they have little real fear of AIDS.

I (DES) examine hundreds of teens each year. I have not yet found one hypersexed heterosexual teen, who sees himself (or herself) at real risk for AIDS. One boy's response to this information was typical, "Yeeoh, bummer. Gotta watch it, huh?" He might have used a condom for his next sexual conquest but he definitely would not change his behavior in any other way.

Teens today hear (the false information) that condoms are the answer, but the majority of teenagers don't consistently use condoms. One student told me, "I'm safe. None of my friends have AIDS." But was she really safe? No. Teenagers may catch HIV, but they take an average of ten years to get sick. By the time they get sick, they are in their mid-twenties; of course, they don't have any friends still in high school.

HIV-positive high schoolers seem perfectly healthy. They don't act sick. They don't feel sick. They don't look sick. They are not sick. In active athletes, HIV stalks high school hallways. In bikinied beauties, HIV lies on sunny beaches. In drunken

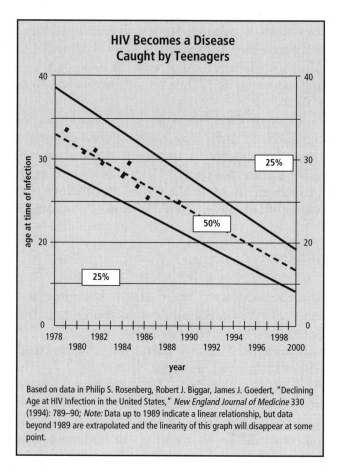

**HIV Becomes a Disease
Caught by Teenagers**

age at time of infection

25%

50%

25%

year

Based on data in Philip S. Rosenberg, Robert J. Biggar, James J. Goedert, "Declining Age at HIV Infection in the United States," *New England Journal of Medicine* 330 (1994): 789–90; *Note:* Data up to 1989 indicate a linear relationship, but data beyond 1989 are extrapolated and the linearity of this graph will disappear at some point.

kids, HIV parties on. Meanwhile, every sex act is a potentially fatal attraction.

Teens may not see it happening. They may think of as a disease of the poor and minorities, but an invisible tidal wave of AIDS is beginning to spill into white, middle-class high schools.

AIDS and Orphans

Millions who suffer the fallout from AIDS are even younger. Some are babies with AIDS; many more are the orphans of

AIDS. Most women who get AIDS are single mothers. It is a hell on earth for a woman to feel the AIDS virus snuffing out her life, while she struggles to care for her young children. She often awakens with the nightmare that she has died. Her children are orphans, fending for themselves. What's worse, she realizes that the nightmare will soon come true.

We are witnessing an epidemic of AIDS orphans. In America more children lose a parent to AIDS than to motor vehicle accidents. In Africa more than *ten million children* will be orphaned by AIDS by the year 2000.

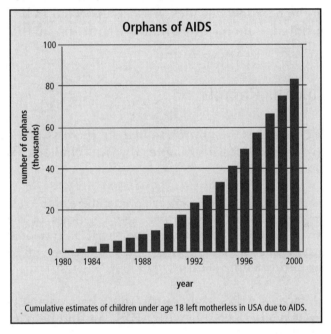

Cumulative estimates of children under age 18 left motherless in USA due to AIDS.

The pain of these AIDS orphans is heart wrenching. Their whole world is falling apart. Often a brother or sister has already died from AIDS. Mom slowly wastes away into a skin-covered skeleton, struggling even to speak.

Mom disappears, off to a graveyard. Sisters and brothers disappear, off to foster homes. Their pain won't disappear. They know the anguish of the African slaves who sang, "Sometimes I feel like a motherless child." It started with the argument, "I can do whatever I want in my own bedroom, so long as it doesn't hurt anybody." Today it is hurting millions—millions of innocent children.

AIDS and the Future

The AIDS epidemic shows no sign of letting up. Even an effective vaccine will take *billions of dollars* and *more than twenty-five years* before beginning to decrease the number of people with AIDS. *Hundreds of millions* will already be dead. World-wide, in the next few decades, AIDS is expected to kill almost three hundred million—more than the entire population of the United States.

AIDS and the Church

AIDS challenges the church to live out its mission of mercy. The *Mayo Clinic Proceedings* notes that this challenge is bigger today than ever before:

> At one time . . . the loving concern of members of the religious community was of considerable help [in times of medical tragedy]. . . . Today, however, . . . the physician cannot always be certain that the patient's religious orientation will be sustaining during a time of crisis.[4]

In the face of AIDS, the church must be a caring community—a place where people with AIDS can find help and hope during their time of trial.

AIDS Is Our Problem

People with AIDS today are only the tip of the iceberg of AIDS suffering. In one way or another, all of us will feel the chill of AIDS.

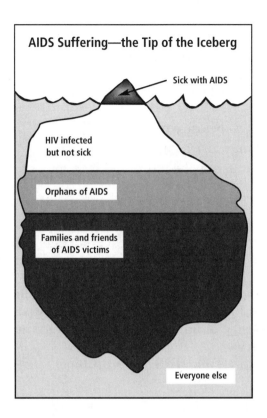

AIDS Suffering—the Tip of the Iceberg

Sick with AIDS

HIV infected
but not sick

Orphans of AIDS

Families and friends
of AIDS victims

Everyone else

None of us can escape being touched. When one person dies, a part of all of us dies. John Donne said:

No man is an island, entire of itself;
    every man is a . . . part of the main. . . .
Any man's death diminishes me,
    because I am involved in mankind.
And therefore never send to know for whom the bell tolls;
    it tolls for thee.[5]

No one can escape the consequences of AIDS. Anyone can catch it:

- A man from a single indiscretion
- A wife from her husband

- A nurse through a drop of blood in a paper cut
- A patient from a transfusion

Those who don't catch AIDS may still be affected:

- A parent may lose a child
- A child may lose a parent
- A Rwandan may be murdered by a mob of hopeless HIV carriers
- A taxpayer will pay higher taxes and health insurance premiums
- Every church will face a great challenge to show the love of Jesus

The Bible says it clearly, "None of us lives a solitary life. None of us dies a solitary death" (Rom. 14:7). Every person is woven into the tapestry of humanity. Each tattered thread mars the entire tapestry.

AIDS affects us all. AIDS is *our* problem.

THIRTEEN

America's Sexperiment

Traditional [i.e., biblical] morality and medical science agree. . . . Abstinence from sexual activity—until a monogamous relationship is established—is the first and most effective line of defense against AIDS.

USA Today, October 1987

On Saturday Lori married the man of her dreams. The next Wednesday should have been the happiest Wednesday of her life, but Lori sat crying in my (DES) office. "What's wrong?" she asked. "What has happened to me?"

She was shivering uncontrollably and wincing from severe genital pain. She held her throbbing head in both hands. Her temperature was 102.3° F. Her groin was covered with weeping, red, burning ulcers—herpes.

Today's pornography always seems to suggest that illicit sex has no consequences. But it isn't true. Herpes is never a pretty picture. Truth in advertising would mean that porn magazines would include gruesome photos of genital herpes. Maybe pornography should also include a warning:

Illicit sex does have consequences—graphic consequences.

Writhing in pain, Lori could barely tolerate an examination. Not only had the virus invaded her genitals, it had spread to her brain, causing encephalitis.

Joe, her churchgoing husband, was a silent herpes carrier. He had never been and never would be sick. Years before, he had sown his wild oats. Now those oats were sprouting in their marriage bed. Lori spent her honeymoon alone in a hospital bed, where she lay feeling guilty, sad, angry, and violated.

Four days earlier, her heart had jumped when she looked toward the front of the church. There stood Joe—handsome, smiling, and hers. Now when he brought flowers to her hospital room, her stomach churned in revulsion. Years later, she still struggled to forgive Joe for her honeymoon herpes.

A measure of forgiveness did come; but, without warning, several times each year, she got a reminder—a herpes relapse. When Lori got pregnant, she suffered constant fear; maybe her baby would get herpes and die or suffer brain damage.

The purity and joy of their sexuality was never the same.

Herpes—the Silent Stalker

You know many people who carry herpes. Herpes lurks in almost every workplace, every family, and every church in America. Up to 60 percent of young adults carry the genital herpes virus.[1] Most (about 75 percent) do not even know they have it. But they can spread the disease, even if they have never had any symptoms.

Yvonne Bryson, of the UCLA School of Medicine, said, "There is a growing spread of an asymptomatic herpes . . . infection. This is a silent infection—you can get it from someone who has no symptoms."

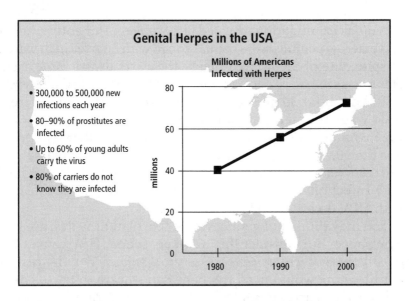

Genital Herpes in the USA

Millions of Americans Infected with Herpes

- 300,000 to 500,000 new infections each year
- 80–90% of prostitutes are infected
- Up to 60% of young adults carry the virus
- 80% of carriers do not know they are infected

People have suffered genital herpes since ancient times, but the sexual revolution of the sixties has produced a raging herpes epidemic. Up to 500,000 new symptomatic cases occur each year. Today herpes is the most common cause of genital ulcers.

In the 1980s herpes carriers started herpes dating clubs to help them find "safe" sexual partners. Unfortunately herpes exists in more than one hundred strains. They caught second and third strains and suffered recurrent attacks from each and every strain. Even worse, people with herpes often carry other STDs, such as HIV, and herpes sores actually help spread HIV. Thus these herpes sex-pairing services actually boosted the spread of herpes and AIDS.

A saying among college students is, "Love may last for only one night, but herpes is forever."

HPV—the Cancer Killer

All through high school and college, Amy had fought off peer pressure and had saved herself for that one special man. She found him and married him. Two years later, she came to see me (DES). She was in tears. "What's wrong with me?" she asked.

A quick examination revealed her problem. Her entire vagina and external genitals were cobblestoned with quarter-inch warts. Despite state-of-the-art treatments, the warts always came back. Her warts seemed as permanent as her blonde hair and blue eyes.

Today, about *30 percent of young adults* carry the venereal wart virus (human papilloma virus or HPV). *From 1969 to 1988, annual doctor visits for genital warts jumped tenfold,* from less than 0.2 million to over 2 million.[2] Today Pap smears from thirteen-year-old girls frequently show dysplasia—a sign of HPV infection. As with HIV and herpes, most people infected with HPV do not even know they have it.

You may think that genital warts, like plantar warts, are just a nuisance. But consider this well-kept secret: HPV causes the *most common female cancer—cervical cancer.* For the rest of her life, Amy would need frequent Pap smears to try to catch cancer in its early stages.

Cervical cancer is not just a nuisance; it is a serial killer. Prior to the AIDS explosion, one authority noted that HPV infection "is the only sexually transmitted disease that commonly kills middle-class American heterosexual women. The fact has been overlooked by everybody in the field."[3]

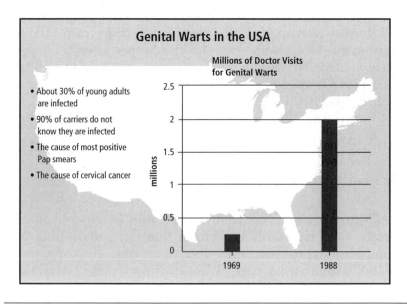

Genital Warts in the USA

Millions of Doctor Visits for Genital Warts

- About 30% of young adults are infected
- 90% of carriers do not know they are infected
- The cause of most positive Pap smears
- The cause of cervical cancer

Doctors rarely tell a woman, *"Your positive Pap smear was caused by HPV, and HPV is an STD."* The woman would be devastated and would need hours of counseling. Instead, doctors simply say, "You have precancerous changes, and you need surgery." Thus millions of women undergo surgery of the cervix, without ever realizing that they are being treated for an STD.

PID—the Secret Sterilizer

Have you ever heard of chlamydia or the disease it causes, pelvic inflammatory disease (PID)? *Scientific American* calls chlamydia "the most *common curable STD* and a *major cause of infertility* in women. . . . [It also] increases the susceptibility of women to *HIV*."[4] *One in twenty middle-class pregnant women* carries a silent chlamydia infection. In newborns, the infection causes *pneumonia* and *premature birth.*[5] One episode of PID leaves 8 percent of women *infertile;* three episodes leave 40 percent *infertile.*[6] Infected women are much more likely to suffer *tubal pregnancies.*[7] Even if the infection is cured with antibiotics one in five women will still suffer years of *chronic pelvic pain.*[8]

PID is the sexual revolution's most secret weapon. Entering a woman during intercourse, chlamydia swim up her uterus

Chlamydia in the USA

The Numbers

- The most common curable STD
- About 4 million new cases each year
- 5% of middle-class women carry silent infections
- 10% of healthy young men carry silent infections

The Results

- A major cause of infertility
- A major cause of ectopic pregnancy
- A major cause of pelvic inflammatory disease (PID)
- Increases risk for transmission of HIV
- Causes premature births
- Causes pneumonia in newborns

into her tubes and abdomen. Within days, the pelvis fills with milky pus. She feels as if her stomach is on fire.

Into her doctor's office she shuffles, doubled over and cradling her burning belly. The jostling from every step unleashes a fiery pain from the inflamed tubes and ovaries. ER nurses sometimes correctly diagnose the problem when the woman enters the ER doing the "PID shuffle."

On internal exam, white pus pours out of the uterus. Even slight movement of the cervix makes the woman jump toward the ceiling—the so called "chandelier sign."

These are the lucky women. With antibiotics they usually get better rapidly. But four out of five women with chlamydia have few symptoms, so they never seek treatment. Over the years, their inflamed tubes scar down into a leathery mass. Sperm and eggs cannot swim up and down the matted tubes.

Many a woman's heart has broken when the doctor has told her that she will never bear children. The doctor will tell her that she has "pelvic scarring," but the doctor will rarely mention where the scarring came from. Her own chlamydia infection will remain a secret, even to herself—the woman from whom it has stolen the joy of childbearing.

The Woodstock Legacy

Where did today's STD epidemic start? Almost everyone agrees; it is a direct result of the so-called sexual revolution.

During three days in August 1969 on a farm near Woodstock, New York, the youth of America declared the founding of the "Woodstock Nation"—the land of sex, drugs, and rock 'n' roll. There a huge crowd of 500,000 middle-class brats camped in a muddy meadow. There they wallowed in free sex, illegal drugs, and angry music. They called it "the dawning of the Age of Aquarius."

They got what they wanted. But did they want what they got?

- They wanted *rock 'n' roll.* Four months later they got a Hell's Angel murdering a Rolling Stones' fan.

- They wanted *drugs*. A year later they got Jimi Hendrix and Janis Joplin—overdosed and dead.
- They wanted *free sex*. For a lifetime they got herpes, genital warts, PID, and a host of other STDs.

At Woodstock no one talked about consequences. "Clap" or "syph" seemed no big deal; you just got a shot of penicillin. If you caught crabs, a little Quell would do ya.

Today the idea of sex without consequences is dead. Today we have herpes—no cure. Today we have PID scarring—no cure.[9] Today we have AIDS—no cure.

Fertility's Bitter Pill

Long ago the consequences of free sex were not so obvious. Long ago there were no Centers for Disease Control, publishing a weekly count of STDs. Long ago there were no tests for syphilis, gonorrhea, or AIDS.

In those ancient times, Canaanite pagan priests ritually raped teenage girls just before their marriage. They hoped that the gods would be pleased and bless the new marriages with many children.[10]

What irony! This so-called *fertility rite* surely infected many new brides with chlamydia. Instead of a fertile womb, they had pelvic scarring. Instead of a large family, they were left barren. One infected priest could rob hundreds of new brides of their chance to bear children.

Many ancient Hebrews privately practiced these pagan fertility rituals. Cultures throughout the ancient Mediterranean practiced similar sex rites. It was so widespread that no other ancient mideastern culture besides the Hebrews seems to have outlawed temple prostitution.

Would the ancient Hebrews add one of these barbaric rituals to the Bible? Would a new bride go to the temple for ritual rape to ensure her future fertility? Would Hebrew temple worship be like others throughout the region, where men paid prostitute priests and priestesses to aid worship?

No. Not one of these rituals is found in the biblical worship guidelines. In fact the ancient Hebrew Bible did not simply ignore these disease-spreading rituals. It specifically forbade them (Deut. 23:17).

How amazing! Again the Bible didn't borrow a disease-spreading practice from the surrounding culture. Again the Bible made a radical break. Again those who obeyed the biblical rules experienced that great promise, "none of these diseases . . ."

America as a Sex Lab

The Bible warns that the seductress of free sex will bring no Age of Aquarius:

> Her lips drip honey,
> and her speech is sweeter than oil.
> But in the end she is a bitter poison,
> as deadly as a double-edged sword.
> Her feet descend to death;
> her steps lead straight to hell.
>
> Proverbs 5:3–5

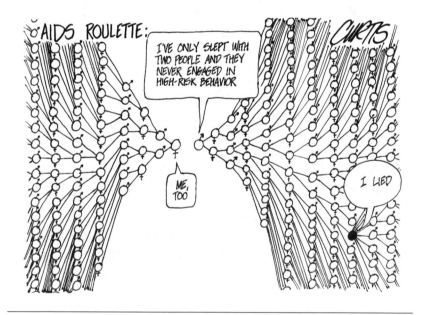

Indeed! America is entering no sexual Aquarius. America is going straight to STD hell. In effect, America has reverted to the sexual practices of the ancient Canaanites. All sorts of sexual perversion now pass as mere *experimentation*. America is a sexual laboratory. Here scientists observe our *experiment in erotomania*. The Centers for Disease Control publishes the weekly results—millions of cases of AIDS, herpes, HPV, gonorrhea, syphilis, PID, chlamydia, and more. These results give scientific proof for the permanent truth of God's precepts.

FOURTEEN

A Woman's Right

Men and women think and feel differently about sex. This is not a sexist idea but merely a scientific observation. Surveys of American college students have found a giant gender gap:

- Sixty of 130 men (versus 0 of 119 women) would "never neglect an opportunity" to have sex.[1]
- Of women, 91 percent felt a one-night stand would leave them "guilty or anxious." Of men, 50 percent thought they would feel "relaxed or satisfied."[2]
- Two-thirds of men admitted to getting "a woman drunk in order to have sex."[3]
- One-third of men had "threatened to leave or to end a relationship if a woman refused to give sex."[4]

At the University of Hawaii, an attractive member of the opposite sex approached students. After a brief introduction, he or she would come right out and ask, "Would you have sex with me tonight?" Not even one woman was interested, but 75 percent of men were more than willing to hop into the sack with a complete stranger.[5]

A Condom for the Heart

In general, men and women have different sexual motives. Women desire intimacy; men desire pleasure. This male attitude is a common reality but it is not right. It is simply one manifestation of humanity's sin problem.

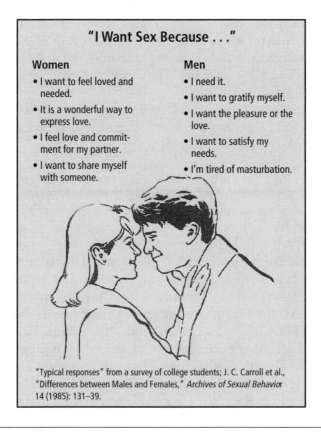

"I Want Sex Because ..."

Women
- I want to feel loved and needed.
- It is a wonderful way to express love.
- I feel love and commitment for my partner.
- I want to share myself with someone.

Men
- I need it.
- I want to gratify myself.
- I want the pleasure or the love.
- I want to satisfy my needs.
- I'm tired of masturbation.

"Typical responses" from a survey of college students; J. C. Carroll et al., "Differences between Males and Females," *Archives of Sexual Behavior* 14 (1985): 131–39.

In casual sex, a man selfishly gives nothing and takes what he wants—physical satisfaction. In casual sex, a woman gives her body but gets nothing in return. After a fleeting moment of intimacy, she finds herself alone again. Her vain attempt to feel close and loved leaves her feeling even more lonely and unloved.

No matter how much society pushes "safe sex," casual sex will never be emotionally safe. No one will ever manufacture a condom for the heart. Saved sex, not safe sex, protects the heart.

Confessions of a Casanova

In relationships many men seek sex but shun commitment. When they do get married, however, most married men do report that sex is "better after marriage."[6]

Today, however, many women have accepted the free-sex lie. They expect little more than dinner and a movie before sex. Finding so many willing casual partners, many men waste decades in casual selfish sex. They miss out on the richness of intimate marital sex.

After finally getting married, Warren Beatty, the man described by *USA Weekend* as a former "quintessential Casanova," described the failures of casual sex:

> My generation paid a big price. . . . It was an amazing opportunity for a generation of people to see that this kind of freedom—or license, if you want a pejorative—is certainly not the answer to happiness.[7]

An "amazing opportunity"? Millions of men and women never needed to experiment with their bodies to make this painful discovery. They already knew that license never ends in happiness. Instead of a sexologist's glossy, trendy paperback, they had followed God's sex manual—the Bible: "Honor marriage, and guard the sacredness of sexual intimacy between wife and husband. God draws a firm line against casual and illicit sex" (Heb. 13:4 *The Message*). God says, "Practice free sex, pay a high price. Save sex for marriage, earn great dividends."

Serial Monogamy—A Serial Killer

Sally was upset. "No way! I don't sleep around. When I'm with a guy, I stick with him." By age thirty-two she had slept with "only four" men. With each man, she had been emotionally involved and sexually faithful. Even so, one of her four "faithful" lovers had left her with a good-bye gift—chronic chlamydia. She would never be able to bear a child.

As Sally did, many people deceive themselves. In their minds, only loose people who have loose sex get STDs. Somehow, loving people with loving sex seem safe. These faithful-till-we-split relationships may feel warm and exciting; but they give only an illusion of safety. In reality they often lead to hassles, heartaches, and herpes. Bacteria and viruses do not check for a couple's emotional commitment. Casual or caring, when it comes to catching STDs, sex is sex.

Remaining hidden and incurable for years, STDs may jump to any new partner. Thus studies have found that your STD risk is *not* determined by your loyalty to each partner. *Your STD risk is determined by your total number of partners during your lifetime.* In sex, there is no safety in numbers.

Former Surgeon General C. Everett Koop once said, "I tell people that when they have sex with someone, they're also having sex with everyone else with whom that person has ever had sex. Naturally if the 'everyone else' is only you . . . you're very well protected from disease . . . and from a lot of other unpleasant surprises as well."[8]

Stand Up and Scream

For centuries women understood how to take control of a sexual relationship. They demanded a trip to the altar before a trip to the bed. In the early twentieth century, 97.5 percent of brides had never had sex with another man. For most newlywed men, their wife was their first sexual partner.[9] If a man wanted sex with a respectable woman, he married her.

Even today 85 percent of American adults still believe that it is always or almost always wrong for teens under sixteen to have sex.[10] Unfortunately parents have failed to convince their children. Almost 40 percent of today's high school boys have had sex with at least four different girls.[11] A century ago most girls would be "sweet sixteen and never been kissed"; *today only a minority of girls will be "sweet sixteen and never had sex."*[12]

Women won the sexual revolution, but what exactly did they win? Every Tom, Dick, and Harry got a trifle. Every Mom, Vick, and Mary got a tragedy.

- Tom dumps his pregnant girlfriend.
- Dick gets a wart or two.
- Harry catches a simple infection.

- Mom becomes a single parent.
- Vick gets cervical cancer.
- Mary becomes sterile from chlamydia.

In effect, the liberated woman has volunteered to be sexually harassed. Dr. James O. Mason, former Director of the Centers for Disease Control, has said, "Sometimes I wonder why the female population doesn't stand up and scream."[13]

A Woman's Right

Women have an inalienable right to keep their virginity until marriage. With this right comes power. Harvard-trained psychiatrist Dr. Keith Ablow notes, "The proper right of women to accept or refuse advances makes them *instant authority figures.* Women can say *no.*"[14]

Think of the power of a chaste woman:

- Thousands of deadly duels have been fought to defend her.
- Trillions of sleepless nights have been lost to yearn for her.
- Hundreds of millions of sworn bachelors have married to obtain her.

Is chastity merely a temporary strategy for immature teens who lack confidence?

"We often encourage students to use abstinence as a temporary strategy if they're not yet confident about negotiating a sexual relationship."

Richard Keeling, M.D.,
Director of the Student Health Service at the University of Virginia

For ages, women have understood that withholding sex gives them incredible power. One virgin told *Glamour* magazine, "Men who only want sex are quickly scared away, and I am left with those who are interested in getting to know me as a person."[15]

But if she becomes, as they say, "sexually empowered," then her true power—the power of her virginity—vanishes. She can not test a man's true intentions. Too many men say, "Why buy the cow, when you get the milk for free?"

In addition to power, a chaste woman also possesses an inner peace:

- She doesn't worry about deciding with whom to have sex.
- She doesn't worry about catching an STD.
- She doesn't worry about giving herpes or HIV to her newborn.
- She doesn't worry about being used for mere physical gratification.

When a woman loses her chastity, she loses her power and loses her peace. It seems no surprise that the so-called winners of the sexual revolution often feel more like victims than victors.

When *Cosmopolitan* surveyed their readers, they found that even Cosmo women had been deeply disappointed by Cosmo's slick, sensual, and selfish sex. The editors noted, "So many readers wrote negatively about the sexual revolution, expressing longings for vanished intimacy, and the now elusive joys of romance and commitment, that we began to sense that there might be a sexual counter-revolution underway in America."[16]

One Woman's Journey

V. Mary Stewart shares her journey to the sexual counter-revolution in her book *Sexual Freedom:*

> I began to see that the need to be always in a sexual relationship with someone really did not have that much to do with the release of sexual tension. Rather, it was a desperate fight against a rarely admitted loneliness and isolation; it was the best (or only) way I knew how to approximate some reassurance that somehow, for a little while anyway there was a semblance of commitment, caring and communication. Very simply, it was an attempt to fill that "God-shaped void" of which Pascal wrote. Over the weeks and months that I still tried to get the best of both worlds, that is, tried to be a Christian and still sleep around, I reached two conclusions. The first was that while I had never had any trouble *attaining* that desired commitment and communication, I was never able to *maintain* it. It was always the same way: A fellow and I would start out with a tremendous euphoric closeness which sooner or later became empty and ritualized. We would go along playing the game for a while, but finally one or the other of us would pull out, determined that next time it would be different. It never was.
>
> The second thing I learned was that feeling isolated has little to do with whether or not one is sharing a bed with someone, or even trying to share a life. I cannot count the nights I have lain awake, sometimes muffling sobs in a pillow, beside a satiated, soundly sleeping male, wondering why I was feeling so alone. It was not that the men in question were doing all the taking and not giving—I did not specialize in relationships like that. Mostly they were people who themselves wanted a real and pretty total relationship. But somehow, just because we were trying to get it all from each other, we ended up having less than we started with, feeling only constraint instead of communication. Somehow we were running the relationship on the wrong fuel.
>
> On the other hand, I will never forget the tremendous liberation I felt the first night I had enough strength in the Lord to say "No" and not feel any need to apologize for it or rationalize it. I remember how good it felt to fall asleep alone, in my own bed, by myself, and how overjoyed I was to wake up in the morn-

ing and confirm that no one was there beside me. I have never felt *less* isolated in my life—then, or ever since.[17]

"NO" is the source of sexual power; "NO" is the password to sexual peace. Women today need encouragement and permission to say "NO."

Men vs. Women		
	Men	**Women**
• Percentage of college men and women admitting to **six or more** sexual partners.	57	19
• Percentage of college men and women who considered **emotional involvement** as only **"sometimes"** or **"never"** necessary before sexual intercourse.	60	15
• Percentage of college men and women who would feel **"guilty or anxious"** after a **one-night stand.**	50	91
• Percentage of college men and women who would **"never neglect an opportunity"** to have sex.	46	0

J. C. Carroll et al., "Differences between Males and Females," *Archives of Sexual Behavior* 14 (1985): 131–39.

Exercising the right to say no truly liberates women. Long ago the Bible stated this eternal principle:

Since we want to become spiritually one with the Master, we must not pursue the kind of sex that avoids commitment and intimacy, leaving us more lonely than ever. . . . Didn't you realize that your body is a sacred place, the place of the Holy Spirit? Don't you see that you can't live however you please, squandering what God paid such a high price for?
1 Corinthians 6:17–20 *The Message*

God made your body a "sacred place." He intended for you to treat your body with dignity and respect. You have a right to chastity. When you exercise your right to say no, then you will know power, purity, and peace.

FIFTEEN

Our Condom Nation

Steve, the local high school star quarterback, entered my (DES) office with confidence. His every move conveyed a cocky machismo. He had come for his yearly sports physical.

I found him in perfect health and I reviewed a few wellness issues:

- Yes, he drove drunk.
- No, he didn't wear a seat belt.
- Yes, he was sexually active—several different girls each week.
- No, he never wore condoms.

He could tell which girls were "clean" just by looking at them. He had no interest in condoms. "I won't buy them," he said. "I won't wear them. I won't even look at them." Once, when a girl insisted that he wear a condom, he "just slipped it off when she wasn't looking."

Six months later, I saw Steve again. He wasn't so cocky this time. Later that week he limped onto the football field for the championship game. He played terribly, and his team lost. Steve and I were the only two people in town who knew the true reason for his miserable performance; Steve was suffering a painful attack of genital herpes.

The Gospel according to the Condom

Sexperts everywhere urge teens, "Be safe. Use a condom." The way they praise condom protection, you might mistake this thin layer of latex for the Great Wall of China. But it isn't working. Despite the hype, many teens tune out the condom evangelists. Among Americans who sleep with multiple partners, only one in six consistently uses condoms.[1]

Even worse, no one has shown that condom education can slow the STD epidemic. Much evidence suggests that it actually boosts the spread of STDs. When the *Medical Tribune* challenged the Centers for Disease Control, the CDC couldn't cite a single good study "demonstrating significant HIV risk reduction due to prevention."[2] The CDC themselves admit: "Behavioral science theory suggests that educational messages about a disease and how it is transmitted will have little impact on behavior change."[3]

USA Today reported a "progressive" Colorado school where they had been handing out condoms for three years. In that time, "The birth rate . . . soared to 31 percent above the national average." In 1992 they expected 100 births to 1,200 students.[4] The condom message had the opposite of the desired effect. It seemed to tell the kids that teen sex was normal and acceptable. They heard the message and they acted on it.

The "safe-sex" message doesn't seem to work for educated adults either. Researchers followed eighty-one college-educated women who visited an STD clinic asking for HIV counseling and testing. Many of these women were at high risk for AIDS, but somehow a negative HIV test gave them a false sense of security. When it came to risky behavior, researchers were stunned to discover that HIV testing and condom counseling had zero effect.[5]

AIDS counseling has also failed to change behavior among gay men[6] and among college students.[7] Researchers at the University of Arkansas found that "although adolescent females have an awareness about AIDS, their behavior [use of condoms] remains unchanged."[8]

But when the sexperts hear the data, they simply reply that the problem is that the education has been too tame. It needs to be more explicit, more intense, and more condom oriented. One author states, "HIV counseling and testing is a critical component of the AIDS prevention effort."[9] Come again? A "critical component" of AIDS prevention remains a method that even the experts themselves admit has failed in multiple studies.

Even teens see the problem. A *USA Weekend* poll found that 63 percent of teens were concerned about the safe-sex message "because it might condone casual sex." *Most teens felt that their teachers were not putting enough emphasis on abstinence.*[10]

Proving this point, in the 1980s the State of Maryland ran a "just say no to sex" high school program. The results: While the national teen pregnancy rate increased 8 percent, teen pregnancies and abortions in Maryland went down.

Surgeon General Dr. C. Everett Koop prophetically stated: "An AIDS education that accepts children's sexual activity as inevitable and focuses only on 'safe sex' will be at best ineffectual, at worst itself a cause of serious harm. . . . Young people should be taught that the best precaution is abstinence."[11]

Maybe we should go even farther. Abstinence is far more than the "best precaution." Let's tell our teens the truth. Abstinence is moral, intelligent, normal, fulfilling, loving, and safe.

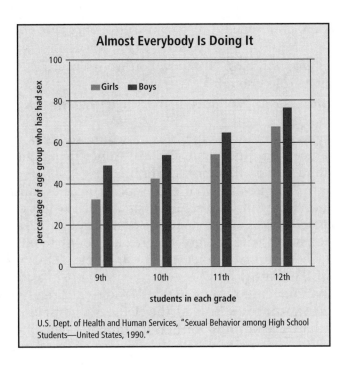

Almost Everybody Is Doing It

percentage of age group who has had sex

▉ Girls ▉ Boys

students in each grade

U.S. Dept. of Health and Human Services, "Sexual Behavior among High School Students—United States, 1990."

Preferences or Values

Some "enlightened" sexologists do sound like they support abstinence. Debra Haffner, executive director of the Sex Information and Education Council of the United States, says, "Parents can tell their children what their values are: 'We think you are too young to have sexual intercourse,' for example."[12]

Maybe that will work. Maybe we should simply tell our kids that they are too young for sex, as we do for makeup or pierced ears. If we express our preferences, maybe they will listen.

But wait a minute. Tell teens that they are "not old enough" for something, and you almost guarantee they soon will be doing it. They will want to *prove* that they *are* old enough. Their parents have one preference; but they have a different preference.

Personal preferences fail, because *preferences are not values.*

- A *preference* says: *"We wish* you would wait for sex until you are old enough."
- A *value* says: "Sex outside marriage is *wrong."*

Personal preferences change on a whim, so teens flounder in this uncertain quicksand. Biblical values never change, so teens stand safe on this moral Gibraltar.

Teens may argue with your preferences, but they must either accept or reject your values. Any hormone-driven guy can wear down a girl who says, "My parents don't think I'm ready *yet."* He will answer, "Sure you are. You're old enough to fall in love. . . . You feel what I feel, don't you? . . . If it doesn't feel right, we can stop." And away they go.

Her parents cared. They meant, "You're not ready yet," to encourage abstinence. Instead, they left her defenseless against wolves that care nothing for her. It's much easier for a girl to say, "No! It's wrong. I won't do it!" She isn't stressed out trying to decide if she is "old enough" yet. She doesn't have to be a debating genius in the back of a Chevy Camaro. The answer to every line is the same. "No. It's wrong."

Mere preferences produce indecision and lead to an STD clinic. Convictions give courage and offer real protection.

Every fall I (DES) do scores of teen sports physicals. At fourteen and fifteen, teens often parrot their parents, "Sex? Not this year. I'm not ready. I'm going to wait." I encourage them and warn them of the dangers of teen sex. But a year later, they sheepishly grin and say something like, "I guess I was ready."

Even in the age of AIDS, when the road to death seems clearly marked, people can refuse to see the road signs. The Bible cautioned against ignoring God's values and following human preferences:

> From a human perspective,
>   there is a road that seems right;
> but its destination is death.
>   Proverbs 14:12

Teens and Sex	
• Median age of **first intercourse** for American boys.	15.5
• Median age of **first intercourse** for American girls.	16
• Percent of sexually active teenage boys who will have **four or more** partners before the age of 17.	40
• Percent of sexually active teens who will catch an **STD each year.**	25

A Culture of Risk

Most teens don't fear death. Teen culture is a bungee-jumping, cigarette-smoking, drag-racing, drug-experimenting, alcohol-bingeing, sex-playing underworld. Teen sex often occurs when teens are so drunk they can barely open a condom package, let alone carefully follow the umpteen essential steps.

This wreckless teen culture remains underground except when it surfaces as an arrest, a car wreck, or a pregnancy. STDs remain especially hidden because teens themselves are often unaware of their own infections. When they do have symptoms, they usually seek treatment without their parents' knowledge.

The Children's Aid Society estimates that *one in every four sexually active American teenagers catches an STD every year.*[13] Thus if a teenager has sex, sooner or later he or she will catch an STD. It's only a matter of time.

Long ago the Bible predicted the fate of a sexual thrill seeker:

> He will die for lack of discipline,
> led astray by his own great folly.
> Proverbs 5:23 NIV

Nothing has changed in almost three thousand years.

The Condom Con

Still, some people feel safe because they always use condoms. They tell us, "I can't have *(name your STD)*. I always wear a condom." We have heard this line over and over from patients testing positive for herpes, chlamydia, HIV, or some other STD.

"Condoms do not offer absolute protection," an AIDS textbook states. "They may be defective, rupture, or come off."[14]

> "There is no such thing as safe sex."
>
> Dack Rambo,
> soap opera star and HIV carrier

"Wait a minute," say the condom backers. "Is it safer to have sex with or without a condom?"

Maybe they are asking the wrong question. What if they asked, "Is it safer to walk through a gun battle with or without a bullet-proof vest?" Of course, it is safer to wear a vest; but why walk through a gun battle in the first place? Bullet-proof vests fail; so do condoms.

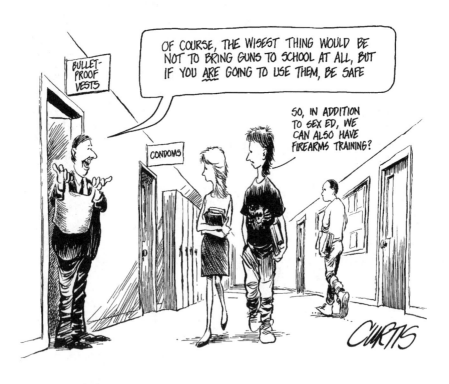

Even before they come out of the package some condoms are leaky. Condom defects are unavoidable, so the FDA approves condom lots where four in one thousand condoms leak.

Family Health International, a family planning agency, studied 850 couples. They found that during marital sex, less than 2 percent of condoms break, but during casual sex, about 5 percent of condoms break. Some highly energetic men break 20 percent of their condoms.[15]

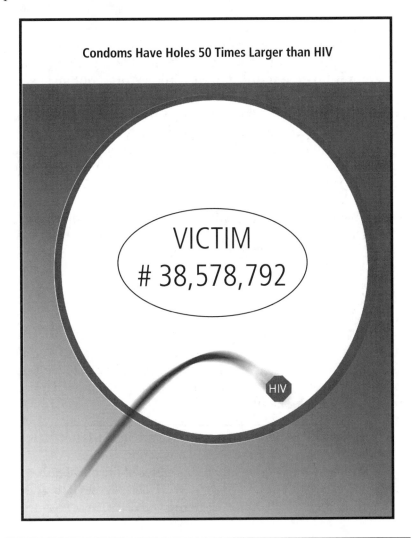

Condoms Have Holes 50 Times Larger than HIV

VICTIM
38,578,792

HIV

Sometimes a woman visits my (DES) office with an embarrassing problem. A condom came off during sex, and she can't find it. The condom is easily removed; but when it comes to STD protection, she might as well have left the condom in her purse.

Dr. Susan Weller of the University of Texas reviewed every study on condoms and STDs. Then she concluded in the journal *Social Science and Medicine:* "Results of HIV transmission studies indicate that *condoms may reduce risk of HIV infection by approximately 69 percent.* Thus efficacy may be much lower than commonly assumed."[16]

Incredible! The world is placing its hope for AIDS prevention in a method that fails about one-third of the time. What if parachutes failed one-third of the time? Would public schools tell our kids, "We know that you are going to jump out of airplanes no matter what we say, so be safe. Use a parachute."

Let's use some common sense. What woman would agree to store toxic waste in a condom stuffed in her genital tract? Can you imagine the Environmental Protection Agency approving condoms for vaginal storage of toxic waste? Ridiculous!

But HIV is as lethal as any toxic waste. Still, our government not only condones placing this toxic waste in condoms; it even advertises it on TV. Sexperts recite their lethal mantra, "Safe . . . Safe . . . Safe . . ." There's nothing safe about it.

Fact-Based Fear

"Stop!" educators object. "What are you trying to do, scare these kids?" Yes. Fear isn't always bad. Fear can be good if it is based on facts. We fear driving off bridges, because we know the fact of gravity. We fear drinking arsenic, because we know the fact of what poison can do.

It is incumbent on all of us to make a frontal assault on the sexual revolution. . . . What was once a matter of morality is today quite literally a matter of life and death.

Dr. Harvey Fineberg,
Dean of the Harvard School of Public Health

STD facts should terrify any teen Juliet speeding toward sex with a turbo-charged Romeo. Teens need to see fact-based fear as a red light, warning, "Stop! Sex outside of marriage can wreck your life. Don't do it! Wait for the green light of marriage."

Marriage—It's Not a Dirty Word

The law requires public sex educators to teach that sex and marriage do go together like a horse and carriage. In 1987 the U.S. Senate passed a law (94 to 2), stating, "All AIDS educational, informational, and preventive materials and activities for school-aged children and young adults shall emphasize . . . abstinence from sexual activity outside of a monogamous marriage."[17] Have the sex educators read this law?

Instead, most sexologists reject this approach. They feel that teaching kids about chastity or marriage involves "value judgments." They say, "Our job is teaching facts not morals. We must respect everyone's values." Thus they flout the congressionally mandated values and replace them with so-called value-free how-to-have-sex education.

One of the U.S. Public Health Service "national health objectives" for the year 2000 was a 50 percent increase in 17-year-old virgins.[18] They didn't come close.

Instead of abstinence, educators crack jokes as they teach teens to slip condoms on bananas. They have kids put condoms over their heads and blow through their noses to produce comical condom coneheads. The idea is to get the kids comfortable with condoms.

They hide the failures of condoms as though they were classified information. For example, an article *for doctors* in *Patient Care* admitted *the condom's "effectiveness against STDs" is only "30–60 percent."* In the same issue they published a patient handout, "Advice for Teenage Girls," stating, *"Using condoms is the only way* to reduce the risk of getting AIDS."[19] What? Wouldn't abstinence work even better? Why weren't the teenage girls given the whole truth? Why just the doctors? Sexperts say they merely teach kids the facts to make good decisions. But they don't give them the facts. Instead, they tell them to trust a condom. Why not the truth? Tell them, "Only a fool trusts a '50:50,' paper-thin latex membrane." Why not the time-proven method? Tell them, "Just say no."

When it comes to drugs, educators understand this concept. They don't tell teens, "Use drugs *safely*." They don't practice *safe* injections of oranges. They don't hand out *safe* drugs. That kind of education would not be *safe;* it would be dangerous. It would only cause a massive drug epidemic. They tell them, "Just say no!" It works for drug education. It works for sex education.

We must take the time to teach teens:

- You are a beautiful creation.
- Your body matters.
- You can take responsibility for your body.
- You don't need to give in to every urge.
- Marital sex is the only safe sex.

Self-respect and self-control—it has never been an easy message. In 1892 Sir William Osler, perhaps the greatest medical doctor since Hippocrates, stated in his classic text *Principles and Practice of Medicine:* "[Chastity] may be a [difficult] condition . . . but it can be borne, and it is our duty [as physicians] to urge this lesson upon young and old who seek our advice in matters sexual."

Over one hundred years later, it remains "difficult" but it "can be borne" and it must be borne, because the lives of a generation are at stake.

When in Rome . . .

Long before Osler, in the ancient Roman Empire, casual sex was also common for both men and women. Masters used slaves for sex. Banquets degenerated into orgies. Men took their marriage vows so lightly that one ancient Roman asked: "Does anyone throw his wife out naked when he happens to find a lover with her, as if he has not enjoyed adultery himself?"[20]

The apostle Paul grew up in the pagan city of Tarsus, where a visitor complained that you couldn't walk in the streets without hearing the panting and grunting of brothel customers.[21] Since Paul grew up surrounded by this cesspool of bawdy sex, you might expect his writings to embrace casual sex; but Paul's writings made a clean break from Roman culture. In effect, Paul urged believers, when in Rome, do *not* do as the Romans: "God wants you to live differently from those around you and to avoid loose sex. Treat your own bodies with dignity and respect. Don't abuse them in lustful passion, as your godless neighbors do" (1 Thess. 4:3–5).

Truly Safe Sex

The Centers for Disease Control clearly states in its "Guidelines for Effective School Health Education": "Sexual relations should occur only in the context of monogamous marriage."[22]
The Bible agrees:

> Drink water from your own cistern,
>   running water from your own well. . . .
> Let her be yours alone,
>   never to be shared with strangers.
> May your fountain be blessed,
>   and may you rejoice in the wife of your youth.
> Proverbs 5:15, 17, 18

God is no sexual killjoy. He made sex for pleasure and pro-creation—not anxiety and STDs. Like a caring Father, he only wants the best for us. He wants us to save sex:

for the best person
at the best time
for the best reason.

SIXTEEN

Spiritual Sexuality

Sex has special meaning. It is not something to be treated casually or without respect.

Alvin Poussaint,
Harvard psychiatrist

"Doctor, what's missing from my life?" Colleen asked. "Jack says he loves me, but I just don't feel it. Every time I try to talk about it, he just shuts me out. He says he's doing what he can. He works hard, and we have a good life: two kids, a nice house. I don't even have to work. What more could I ask for? Maybe that should be enough. He is a good provider . . . but around him, I feel like I don't exist. He watches football, he reads the newspaper, but he hardly notices me—except at night when he turns off the TV. Then he hugs and kisses me, but it's only because he suddenly wants sex. He doesn't care about me. It's like a ten-minute drill—get undressed, brush teeth, use the toilet, do it, and go to sleep. It leaves me cold. Sometimes I wish he would get a mistress, just so

I could get a break. My friends tell me to dump Jack . . . I don't know. Maybe I just need some Prozac."

Colleen and Jack clearly had problems. Both grew up in emotionally cold homes where no one talked about sex. Neither had ever seen their parents hug, kiss, or even share a tender word. Colleen's mother had passively communicated that ladies simply put up with sex and nice girls never enjoy it.

Colleen found sex dirty and disgusting. Jack saw sex simply as his right and her duty.

Sometimes sex seems to give birth to more problems than babies. Some might even feel like sex is somehow the devil's dirty trick. Many early church fathers made this mistake. They wrongly accepted dualism, a Greek philosophy that the soul was good but the body was bad. Since the body was evil, truly "spiritual" people beat their bodies, took vows of poverty, and even wore irritating wool underwear. Sex involved the body, so sex was bad. Sex was a weakness for those not "spiritual" enough to resist temptation. Permanent celibacy was for spiritual giants.

Scripture contradicts these strange ideas. God created both soul and body and God declared all of his creation "good." Sex has always been a part of the divine design for human dignity.

Sex as Sacred

A patient of mine (DES) once came for treatment of gonorrhea. He was a well-known businessman in the community going through a midlife crisis. One day he found himself, for the first time in his life, in a hotel room with a prostitute. After he paid her, she laid down the rules. "I'm Jane. You're Joe. No small talk. Wear this condom. Kiss me anywhere you want except my mouth."

In a strange twist of logic, she gave up her sex organs but saved her lips for a relationship that would involve not only her body, but also her soul. She was allowing her body to be used as a pleasure toy, but something in her soul cried out, "Save something for the soul." So she made this vain attempt to protect her soul.

God made sex sacred and good. When sex is part of a loving marriage, both partners don't need to hold back anything. They are free to enjoy and give themselves completely to each other.

In this kind of sex, we can experience blessing in our everyday lives. Thus sex can be a spiritual sacrament.[1] Sex can be the union of two bodies and two souls, both experiencing the blessing of God. God created sex to be a natural act of worship. God wants us to live in his presence always, even during sex.

Because couples often suffer sexual hang-ups, they may find communion with God during sex unthinkable. One way to test if you are comfortable with both your spirituality and sexuality is to ask yourself if you can freely begin sex with the prayer, "Lord, for what we are about to receive, we give thanks." In this kind of spirituality, two people can experience the superlative in sex—a union of both their bodies and their souls.

The Illusion of Romantic Love

Today few people think of spirituality when they think of sex. Instead, most people think of romance—where a fairy-tale prince sweeps a fairy-tale princess into a fairy-tale bed of perpetual passion. But real life is never a fairy tale. The gravity of time always pulls the "happily-ever-after" fantasy down to earth. When the roses of romance wilt, many a lover is left disappointed and disillusioned.

We all have a hole in our hearts. Our souls long for completeness, so the illusion of romantic love appeals to us. The heart may try to fill its hole with a romantic lover. But when the lover has given all, the soul still cries out for more. Lovers always disappoint, so the soul must search for another lover. If we keep this up, our heartache never ends.

Romance is an invitation to take the plunge into LOVE. Going no deeper, romance becomes mere lust. At some point, suddenly the soul feels used and violated.

Still, for many people, even seemingly religious people, the closest that they get to a spiritual experience is sex. In sex, they can scarcely distinguish soul and body. Those few magic moments of electric excitement can bring a false sense of spiritual wholeness. M. Scott Peck relates: "It is because [sex] is a spiritual experience of sorts that so many chase after it with a repetitive, desperate kind of abandon. Often, whether they know it or not, they are searching for God."[2] Romance seeks to fill the heart's hole with a human lover; but the hole is as wide and as deep as God himself. Only God can fill it.

Two stunning bodies devoted to sexual gratification will not find soul satisfaction. The constant couplings and uncouplings of Hollywood's stars prove the emptiness of selfish sex. Too often people expect soul satisfaction from the sparks of heart-pounding sex. Like a lightbulb, these incandescent feelings quickly burn out. Passion's light goes out. The heart's hole remains a dark void.

Conflict—Rocky Road to Real Intimacy

Remember Jack and Colleen? Early in their marriage they had found their differences intriguing. But soon Jack's matter-of-fact thinking began to conflict with Colleen's more emotional approach.

Colleen expected flowers and kisses; Jack thought it was enough to bring home a paycheck. Colleen wanted to talk about their day; Jack just wanted to relax and forget his work. Colleen wanted to take the scenic route; Jack would try to save a minute and drive right through the industrial section of town.

Every time a conflict came up, they were shocked to see that they had married someone who didn't see the world in a "normal" way. They would fight and never find resolution. If they opened up about their feelings and expectations, they faced conflict and rejection. Soon they both decided to avoid opening up. That way they could avoid fighting. They became emotional islands separated by oceans of fear and resentment.

But Jack and Colleen had failed to realize that only through opening up and working through their conflicts could they experience any closeness. They might tolerate each other but they would never find intimacy.

Intimacy requires transparency and a willingness to open up. Paul wrote in Romans 12:9 that this kind of LOVE was "without make believe." Openness always brings some conflict, but this conflict can lead to intimacy. The sparks of conflict are signs of life in a marriage. The yawns of boredom suggest that no one cares, and love has evaporated.

Many sue for divorce because of "incompatibility." What they fail to realize is that everyone is incompatible with everyone else. No truly compatible couple has ever existed. We are all different. We all have different wants. We all have different styles. We all have different expectations. We all have different joys. We all have different trials. We all have different temptations. We all have different differences. Believe it or not, incompatibility is actually one of the purposes of marriage. It is through our differences, conflicts, and resolutions that we grow spiritually and learn tolerance, love, and forgiveness.

Marriage—A Spiritual Journey

The road of sexual spirituality does not start on an orgasmic mountaintop. Instead, it winds through the valleys of everyday life. That is why the Bible does not call the spiritual life a mystical *high* but instead an everyday *walk*. Only those who have chosen this grueling *walk* can experience the mystical heights of true spiritual sexuality.

Adolf Guggenbuhl-Craig sums up why so many couples become confused about healthy sexuality in marriage. "People are continually being taught by psychiatrists, psychologists, marriage counselors, etc., that only happy marriages are good marriages, or that marriages *should* be happy."[3] Marriage, however, is a spiritual journey; and spiritual journeys aren't joyrides to Nirvana. Spiritual journeys are hikes through the canyons, deserts, and jungles of real life. "This is why [marriage] is so filled with highs and lows; it consists of sacrifices, joys, *and* suffering. . . ."[4]

Most "totally in love" couples enter marriage thinking at the outset that romantic love will last forever and that it will always be enough. But romantic love alone is never enough.

If, instead, marriage becomes a spiritual journey along the streams of LOVE, partners can explore the heights and depths of spiritual sexuality. Marriage can provide great delight as a waterfall rushing down the mountains of romantic ecstasy. Marriage can also provide deep satisfaction as a river flowing through the fertile valleys of a meaningful life. Those who travel this spiritual journey can say to each other:

> Grow old along with me!
> The best is yet to be,
> The last of life, for which the first was made.
> Robert Browning

SEVENTEEN

The Secret of Great Sex

There is only one answer for any marriage or any vital relationship. That is to exchange that dividing wall of hostility for the cross of Christ. It is to stop all demands that the other change. It is to die daily to self, to continually ask the Lord, "What in me is contributing to the breakdown of this marriage? . . . What is there in me that needs to die?"

John and Paula Sandford,
The Transformation of the Inner Man

When Colleen and Jack finally talked openly about their relationship, it turned out that they both wanted a return to the sizzling passion of their honeymoon. Back then, just the sight of him made her heart warm with desire. Even Jack admitted that sex was much better in the "old days."

What could they do?

They could read the latest sex manuals. They could make an appointment with the wildest sex therapist. They could attend the most popular sex seminars. If they did, they would fail. Instead, they could use the method tried by millions and found true for centuries.

Love

Jesus offered the world's most effective marriage seminar ever. Jesus summed up his secret formula in a single word: *agape* or LOVE. LOVE means commitment, care, respect, tolerance, and forgiveness. LOVE puts the cuddle in the snuggle and the zest in the nest. "Love never fails" (1 Cor. 13:8).

LOVE is not the ush and gush of romance novels. LOVE is not what the Beetles sang, "All we need is love." LOVE is not the Hollywood starlet's, "He, like, makes me feel things that, like, are so cool."

Aldous Huxley lamented, "Of all the worn, smudged, dog's-eared words in our vocabulary, 'love' is surely the grubbiest, smelliest, slimiest. . . . It has become an outrage to good taste and decent feeling, an obscenity which one hesitates to pronounce."[1]

Why has *love* become such a worthless word? Because we have lost God's definition, the world teems with a million wrong definitions.

God defines real LOVE as when you:

> LOVE your neighbor as yourself.
> Jesus Christ, circa A.D. 30

From birth we are all experts at loving ourselves. We seek food for ourselves. We seek safety for ourselves. We seek significance for ourselves. Real LOVE is that same desire to satisfy and please someone else. Romance says, "What can I get?" LOVE says, "What can I give?"

A love that says, "I love you because you make me happy," will fail. It cannot last, because no lover can *always* make you happy. True LOVE says, "I love you even when you make me unhappy." That kind of love can last and grow.

Francis of Assisi prayed for this LOVE:

> O Divine Master, grant that I may not so much seek
>   to be consoled as to console,
>   to be understood as to understand,
>   to be loved as to love. . . .

This is the only kind of LOVE that would transform Colleen and Jack's marriage.

Is LOVE a Universal Value?

Today there is a widespread myth that all philosophies and religions are basically the same. College professors boldly state that all religions teach love, respect, and commitment. TV commentators note the common values of all religions.

This myth is commonly repeated, but is it true? Is this universalism a product of investigation or ignorance? Of facts or fads? Let's look.

The Hindu and Love

Robert Johnson, author of the book *He,* was one day walking in India with a Hindu holy man. Johnson stopped and gave money to a beggar. The guru stopped and scolded him for meddling with the beggar's karma. Johnson replied that he was not doing it for the beggar. He did it for himself. The guru changed his mind; if the motive was purely selfish, then giving to the poor might be okay.

This thinking sounds strange to those brought up in a Christian culture, but it makes perfect sense to a Hindu. In Hinduism and Buddhism only the spiritual world is real. The material world is merely illusion. Spiritual growth requires detachment from the material world and escape to the spiritual world. LOVE for others has nothing to do with spiritual growth.

In his book *Myths to Live By,* Joseph Campbell extolled the myths of Eastern religions as sources of spiritual truth. On the subject of love, however, he could not find even a single Eastern myth with the theme of love. Thus, late in life, finding the Eastern view incomplete, he abandoned it.

The Materialist and Love

On the other end of the spectrum are the religions of Marxists (dialectical materialism) and humanists (evolutionary materialism). Today's intellectual elitists follow the religion of material-ism. For them only the physical world is real. The spiritual world is illusion. They cannot discuss the spiritual life, for they do not even believe in the spiritual realm. Love is not real. Love is merely a splash of brain chemicals designed to trick animals (that is, people) into mating, reproducing, and passing on their genes.

In this world only the fittest survive. There is no room for sacrificial love. No one should help weak people, because then they might pass on "inferior" genes. Materialists exist to dom-inate and to pass on their own "superior" genes.

The consistent materialist cannot love his neighbor, for his neighbor is just another animal, a competitor in the fight for survival.

The Christian and Love

Jesus recognized that both the physical and the spiritual are real and good. We live the spiritual life right here in the mate-rial world by giving and receiving tangible LOVE.

LOVE is the one great truth unique to Christianity. Mohammed taught judgment, not love. Buddha taught escape, not love. Con-fucius taught conformity, not love. Jesus taught LOVE.

In Islam God is remote and inaccessible. Allah is so far removed that no human could ever be in relationship with him. Only the Bible reveals to us, "God is LOVE" (1 John 4:16).

Jesus called God, "Daddy,"[2] and taught that we are his chil-dren. Jesus called us to an intimate relationship with the Cre-ator of the universe. Jesus also calls us to live in that same LOVE relationship with others.

When people blandly state, "I believe in a god of love," often they are trying to contrast their god of love with the God of the Bible. But they did not come up with the concept of a loving god themselves. They got it from the Bible. What they are really say-ing is this, "I believe in [part of] the God revealed in the Bible."

LOVE is the greatest revelation of history. Jesus did not derive LOVE from other Middle Eastern cultures. He did not observe LOVE in the totalitarianism of the Romans. He did not find LOVE in the Platonism of the Greeks. He did not derive LOVE from the eroticism of the Gentiles. He did not see LOVE in the legalism of the Pharisees.[3]

LOVE was a revelation from God himself. LOVE has no other explanation. LOVE proves that God himself is responsible for the teachings of the Bible.

Porcupines and Love

This LOVE does not come naturally to anyone. We are all porcupines. We all have irritating spines—unlovable and even despicable qualities. People who get close to us always get poked. We all irritate our friends. We all hurt our family. We all let down our neighbors.

In any and every relationship, only LOVE can overlook and heal our relational wounds. C. S. Lewis said:

> There is something in each of us that cannot be naturally loved. It is no one's fault if they do not so love it. . . . You might as well ask people to like the taste of rotten bread or the sound of a mechanical drill. . . . All who have good parents, wives, husbands, or children may be sure that some times and perhaps at all times, in respect of some one particular trait or habit, they are receiving [LOVE]. They are loved not because they are lovable but because Love Himself is in those who love them.[4]

LOVE loves not because of . . . but in spite of. Intimacy means that every day I bump into your porcupine spines, but I LOVE you anyway. When I (DES) married Diane, our pastor shared some great advice. "Every day of your marriage," he said, "something will happen that if you decide to dwell on it, it could lead to divorce."[5]

Successful marriage is not ignoring our spouse's faults. Marriage success means learning to LOVE *in spite of* all the faults we see. Romance loves *because of* . . . Romance says, "I love you *because* you are beautiful. I love you *because* you are so caring. I love you *because* you make me feel good." LOVE says,

"I LOVE you *in spite of* your wrinkles. I LOVE you *in spite of* your carelessness. I LOVE you *even though* you frustrate me."

God LOVES us *in spite of* our faults, *in spite of* our desires to live life without him, *in spite of* our failures to LOVE. This is the great truth of God's LOVE. We do not earn it. We cannot deserve it. In fact God's LOVE means that he is overlooking and forgiving all of our faults. We can LOVE because we have been LOVED so much. We can LOVE because he has forgiven all our sins.

Jesus once overwhelmed a prostitute with forgiveness for her many sins. She responded by bowing low, pouring perfume on his feet, wiping his feet with her hair, and kissing his feet. A self-righteous religious leader was disgusted by this prostitute's display of affection.

Jesus replied, "She LOVES much, because she has been forgiven much. But someone who has been forgiven little, will LOVE little" (Luke 7:47).

We have been forgiven much. That is why we can LOVE much. That is why we can LOVE as God LOVES.

> LOVE is patient. Love is kind. . . . LOVE is not self-seeking. . . .
> LOVE keeps no record of wrongs. . . . LOVE always protects, always
> trusts, always hopes, always perseveres.
>
> 1 Corinthians 13: 4–6

This kind of LOVE loves *in spite of*. This is a supernatural LOVE—a LOVE from God.

Spiritual Oxygen

Men and women often neglect LOVE. Jack would never experience great sex as long as he insisted that Colleen "service" his needs. As long as he insisted on *getting,* he would *get* little.

A sex-centered man, he got little out of sex because he focused on himself instead of on Colleen. Sexually frustrated, his angry explosions boosted his blood pressure and aggravated his angina.

Dr. Carl Jung diagnosed the source of Jack's frustration: "It arises from his having no love, but only sexuality."[6] Jack had never heard that any other type of love existed. He had no idea that sex could involve anything more than self-gratification.

Countless couples feel trapped in loveless marriages. The only love they know is sexual—something pictured in paperback novels and popular movies. They are never satisfied because sex without LOVE smothers the soul.

LOVE is spiritual oxygen. Without it your soul will suffocate. Dr. Smiley Blanton notes:

> For more than forty years I have sat in my office and listened while people of all ages and classes told me of their hopes and fears. . . . As I look back over the long, full years, one truth emerges clearly in my mind the universal need for love. . . . They cannot survive without love; they must have it or they will perish.[7]

Only LOVE can breathe life into the dying soul.

Give Me or Giving

Couples without LOVE are frustrated. They have extramarital affairs, but their frustrations only increase. They fight and never forgive, so sex becomes lifeless and even repulsive. One woman in a loveless marriage said that sex with her husband felt like being raped by a "mechanical gorilla."

These couples often head off to a sex therapist who may give them sex exercises. These exercises may produce temporary relief but they usually treat only symptoms and do not get at the root problem—lack of LOVE.[8]

Psychoanalyst Erich Fromm felt that this lack of LOVE was the root of all psychological problems:

> The injunction, "Love thy neighbor as thyself," is the most important norm of living and . . . its violation is the basic cause of unhappiness and mental illness. . . . Whatever complaints . . . the patient may have, whatever symptoms he may present, are rooted

in his inability to love if we mean by love a capacity for the experience of concern, responsibility, respect and understanding of another person and an intense desire for that other person's growth. Analytic therapy is essentially an attempt to help the patient gain or regain his capacity for love. If this aim is not fulfilled, nothing but surface changes can be accomplished.[9]

Men particularly tend to think that sex alone can nourish a relationship. Orgasm for men can be a fairly mechanical act. For a woman, climax is much more complex. She is not a robot. Just pushing certain buttons will not set off bells and whistles. Dr. Max Levin notes that unselfish LOVE is necessary for great sex.

It is obvious, then, that maturity is a prerequisite for a happy marriage. In the immature state of infancy there is no obligation to give. The infant receives; he is not expected to do anything else. The success of a marriage will depend in great degree on the extent to which the partners have outgrown their infantile dependency and achieved the capacity to assume responsibility, to wish more to give than to receive.[10]

Centuries before Colleen and Jack drifted apart, the Bible noted the need for this kind of maturity.

When I was a baby, I used to talk baby talk and think baby thoughts. But when I grew up, I matured and gave up baby things. . . . This maturity is about faith, hope, and LOVE; of these three, the greatest is LOVE.

1 Corinthians 13:11, 13

The prodigal son discovered that the immature give-me life never satisfies (see Luke 15:11–32). He left home and ran off to a land far removed from his father's values. There he partied away his inheritance. But his give-me scramble left him unhappy and penniless. He hit bottom in one of life's pig pens, where even the hog slop looked tasty.

His heart longed for the LOVE of his father's house. There his needs had always been met. Maybe his father's "horrible religious inhibitions" were not as bad as he had once thought.

Maybe there was a relationship between giving LOVE and receiving blessing.

When he was a child, he had an immature give-me attitude. When he had grown up, he had a mature thoughtfulness. "Make me a servant," he said.

The Importance of Climax

The largest survey of American sexuality extensively probed the sex lives of Americans. One result surprised many. Conservative Protestant women were most likely to reach orgasm every time. One newswriter was startled because these women reminded her of "church bake sales and antiabortion rallies,"[11] not red-hot sex. The researchers themselves noted:

> [These results] seem surprising because conservative religious women are so often portrayed as sexually repressed. . . . The popular image of straitlaced conservative Protestants . . . may be a myth at least as it pertains to sex. . . . Perhaps conservative Protestant women firmly believe in the holiness of marriage and of sexuality as an expression of their love for their husbands.[12]

Indeed, most Christian wives do not fit Hollywood's stereotype icebergs. Some may, but most experience LOVE and terrific joy in orgasmic sex.

Without LOVE, people find marriage restrictive and empty. One in three American women report that they lack interest in sex. One in four have had long-term difficulties in reaching orgasm.[13] Women who rarely climax are three times more likely to be unhappy.[14]

Unfortunately, some men are Victorian dinosaurs, who think that "real ladies don't enjoy sex" and "nice girls don't climax." This selfish attitude looks and feels nothing like LOVE. A woman needs a man who will listen to her sexual needs. She needs emotional closeness. She needs to feel special. She needs to be cared for, not just in the bedroom, but also in the kitchen.

Many husbands and wives could benefit from seeing a good counselor or reading a good book about the sexual response of a woman. With a little information, a few muscle exercises, and a cooperative husband, many women who have never experienced orgasm can easily and often reach climax. One Christian counselor reported that 96 percent of couples who had gone through his premarital counseling had experienced "definite orgasm during marital intercourse."[15] (If you wish more information on this subject, we recommend Tim and Beverly LaHaye, *The Act of Marriage* [Grand Rapids: Zondervan, 1976], and Ed and Gaye Wheat, *Intended for Pleasure*, 3d ed. [Grand Rapids: Revell, 1997]).

Still, orgasm isn't the beginning and end of sex. Many women never climax yet they find sex very satisfying. They can bask in the glow of LOVE's fireplace. They don't necessarily need flashing fireworks.

Unfortunately many sexologists mislead couples to believe that "the big O" is the main goal of all sex. They tout orgasm as a right for women and duty for men. Under this pressure, large numbers of women actually fake orgasm just to "get it over with." When it doesn't happen every time, men may feel inadequate and women may feel cheated.

But orgasm is not the main reason for sex. According to the Bible, God designed sex as a beautiful expression of LOVE between a man and his wife (1 Cor. 7:3–5).[16]

Marriage—the School of Love

If LOVE predominates, even women who have never experienced orgasm can experience greater and greater satisfaction from sex. In fact if a woman communicates her physical desires and if her husband responds in LOVE, she is likely to suddenly and unexpectedly discover the joy of climax. Even if she rarely climaxes, when sex expresses LOVE, both partners can experience a deep satisfaction in their souls.

Someone has said: "The cure for all the ills and wrongs, the cares, the sorrows and the crimes of humanity, all lie in one word LOVE. It is the divine vitality that everywhere produces and restores life. To each and every one of us it gives the power of working miracles if we will."

The Bible applies the LOVE miracle to marriage:

> The marriage bed must be a place of mutuality—the husband seeking to satisfy his wife, the wife seeking to satisfy her husband. Marriage is not a place to "stand up for your rights." Marriage is a decision to serve the other, whether in bed or out.
>
> 1 Corinthians 7:3–4 *The Message*

The secret of great sex is:

> not grabbing, but giving;
> not me first, but you first;
> not technique, but LOVE.

PART 4

EMOTIONAL
WHOLENESS

EIGHTEEN

The Spirit-Mind-Body Link

Hiding behind her mother's skirt and shivering like a panicked puppy, Helen Seibert had changed dramatically from the girl I (SIM) had recently seen for her prekindergarten physical. What had scared her so?

Her mother answered my inquiring look: "Doctor, Helen has been vomiting every day for six weeks. Nearly everything I give her comes up. She began to vomit the day after Labor Day."

That day had been Helen's first day of school. Helen lived far up Turtle Creek. With few neighbors, she had spent most days happily playing alone in her family room or in the woods.

Suddenly school had thrust her into a frightening new world—the "big kids" on the bus, the hustle in the hallways, the rules of her new teacher. Most frightening of all, Mom and Dad were missing from this new world. Stress signals pulsed from her brain to her stomach. Her stomach churned out acid and clamped off its outlet. The excess acid had nowhere to go but up.

Every September we see a few of these cases, but Helen was worse than most. She looked weak and pale and she had lost several pounds. Usually we just reassure the children and parents. We encourage parents to give the children extra emotional support. We encourage the kids to stick with school. Soon they adjust and do well.

The Stress Mess

Stress can also make adults ill. Jane came to my (DES) office obviously overstressed. Five minutes into her health history, she had reviewed the previous two months—the worst two months of her life. She had lost her job. Her husband had left her. Her daughter had gotten into trouble at school. The IRS was auditing her small business. . . . On and on it went.

Finally, I got a word in edgewise and asked her what had brought her to seek medical attention. "I got some stomach flu," she said. "I just can't seem to shake it. For the past week, I've had nonstop diarrhea."

She wanted nerve pills, sleeping pills, stomach pills, or even an antibiotic. She was sure that a pill would cure her. I knew her problem lay deeper than her stomach, but it took a lot of convincing for her to try an alternative prescription. I outlined a different treatment—a regimen of prayer, worship, and counseling. I prayed with her, and we reviewed our plan to help her cope with her life.

After two weeks, she returned for a follow-up visit. "Doctor," she said, "you surprised me when you wouldn't prescribe medication. But you were right. I was overreacting to stress. I still have more stress than I want, but at least the diarrhea's gone."

As long as stress exists, doctors will have plenty of patients. Elaine got migraines "ever since that lousy boyfriend dumped me." Her ex-boyfriend's diabetes spiraled out of control because the breakup kept him from studying for "that ridiculous math test." His teacher's arthritis flared up while grading those "terrible test papers."

A mind upset makes a body sick. With every passing year, researchers find more and more ways that the mind *(psyche)* produces sickness in the body *(soma)*—hence the term *psychosomatic* illness.

Contrary to popular opinion, psychosomatic diseases are not "all in your head." Tension in the mind often triggers or worsens asthma, infections, heart attacks, diabetes, arthritis, and a host of other conditions. Obviously these physical ailments are not merely "in your mind."

Stress—Nothing to Sneeze At

Throughout human history, infection caused most disease and death. At the dawn of the third millennium, health enemy number one is stress (both spiritual and mental). The American Academy of Family Physicians estimates that two-thirds of doctor visits are for "stress-related conditions."[1]

Maybe you have noticed that you often catch a cold after a very stressful week. Scientists have also wondered about the relationship of stress to the common cold. Dr. Sheldon Cohen did an experiment on four hundred volunteers in Salisbury, England. Would you have used a week of vacation to volunteer for this experiment?

1. First, he used psychological tests to determine the current stress levels of the volunteers.
2. Then he squirted cold viruses up their noses.
3. Next, Dr. Cohen put them in quarantine and watched to see who got sick.

Both the high- and low-stress groups were otherwise almost identical:

- They were similar ages.
- They experienced the same weather.
- They lived in the same buildings during the experiment.
- They ate the same food.

In several days, however, the high-stress group began to look very different. They had more red noses, more raspy voices, more watery eyes, and more deep coughs. Nearly twice as many of them had caught colds. By weakening their infection-fighting cells, stress had left them much more susceptible to the common cold.[2]

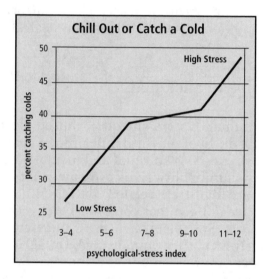

Next time you catch a cold, evaluate your own stress level. Maybe your body is telling you that, when it comes to stress, enough is enough.

The Spiritual Dimension

Through its vast nerve network, the brain "reaches out and touches" every other organ in the body. Thus abnormal brain chemistry influences chemistry throughout the body. The field of psychosomatic medicine is devoted to studying how these chemical interactions are related to health and disease.

Unfortunately most scientists go no further. Scientists generally view humans merely as complex lab animals. To them, people are merely chemicals and chemistry. To them, a psychological problem is merely abnormal brain chemistry. Fix the brain chemistry, fix the problem.

But people are more than chemicals and chemical reactions. People are spiritual beings. What separates humanity from the animals is not the ability to reason. It is not the ability to use tools. People are not merely a few genes separated from chimpanzees. No. We are spiritual at our very nature. Our spirituality is what the Bible calls the "image of God." The spiritual dimension is what separates us from dogs, monkeys, and lizards.

A patient may come to the doctor with a complaint of constant tiredness. Her thyroid is normal. She is not anemic. Her blood sugar is normal. She is surprised to hear that her problem is not just physical. It is not just psychological. At its root, it is spiritual.

She is about to lose her job, so she worries: *How can we afford Christmas presents? How will I find a new job? How will I pay the mortgage?* Her worries go on and on. She reads her Bible, "Trust in the Lord, and He will give you the desires of your heart" (Ps. 37:4). But still she worries. She even feels guilty for worrying. She has an upset spirit. Her spirit is not at peace with God. Her spirit is not at peace with others. Her spirit is not at peace even with her own soul.

Her upset spirit is leading to an upset mind. Her upset mind is firing SOS messages throughout her body. Her glands release stress hormones. These hormones keep her awake at night and stress her body during the day. That is why she is constantly tired. If she does not deal with the root spiritual problem, these chemicals may cause a stroke, a painful arthritis attack, or something even worse.

The Spirit-Mind-Body Cycle

How can spiritual unrest lead to strokes, heart attacks, bleeding ulcers, neck spasms, and even cancer?

Spirit

- Your soul is born with a need to know and experience God. Without this intimate connection, your spirit is in chaos and longs for peace.
- Then comes stress, such as loss of a loved one, loss of a job, or the pain of rejection. This external stress may disrupt your illusion of internal peace and make you aware of your soul's inner chaos.

Mind

- Your brain interprets this unrest as fear, anxiety, worry, anger, or other emotions.
- Through its nerve network, the brain sends alarm signals throughout your body.

Body

- Without asking your permission, your glands release adrenaline, cortisone, insulin, and other stress hormones.
- Every organ becomes overexcited. Blood vessels constrict, the heart speeds up, muscles twitch, and toxins build up in the blood.

In short, you are "stressed out." If this continues for years, your body will literally wear out. All the so-called stress vitamins in the world will not protect you.

Of course, short-term stress reactions are essential and do not lead to chronic disease. If a prowler breaks into your house, a sudden burst of adrenaline stimulates your muscles, dilates your pupils, and puts your mind on alert. You are ready for "fight or flight." This response is not only needed. It may even save your life.

But what if every day your spirit is not confidently resting in the peace of God? Then you may constantly worry about imaginary prowlers lurking in the shadows. Day in, day out, your body stays on red alert. This constant adrenaline rush will drive you down the road to a serious disease.

Spiritual problems may seem purely ethereal but they have many physical results. An upset spirit (*pneuma*) upsets the mind *(psyche)*, and this harms the body *(soma)*. Maybe we need a new term—the *pneumo-psycho-somatic* illness.

The Body's Response

Spiritual *(pneuma)* unrest produces emotional *(psyche)* upset, affecting the body *(soma)* in three ways:

1. Changing Blood Flow
- For example, when you are *embarrassed,* the blood vessels in your cheeks dilate and you blush.
- *Anger* can lead to the spasm of brain arteries and a migraine headache.

2. Changing Secretions
- Remember your *fear* when you first spoke to a large group of people? Alarm messages shot from your brain to your salivary glands, and they stopped secreting saliva. Your mouth felt like it was painted with rubber cement.
- Long-term fear *(anxiety)* may stimulate stomach acid, allow bacteria to invade the stomach lining, and lead to an ulcer.

3. Muscle Spasms
- When you *worry,* your muscles tend to spasm and hurt. That is why worriers suffer so much from back and neck spasms.
- *Depression* often causes multiple irritable trigger points in the muscles. When these trigger points go into spasm, a person suffers the chronic pains of fibromyalgia.

Once a couple sought my (DES) care because muscle spasms were about to end their three-month-old marriage. I greeted them and asked what they had come for. There was a long pause, while they both fidgeted nervously.

Finally, Sue began, "Doctor, please, you've got to help us. Jim wants a divorce."

They had my attention.

It turned out that every time they had tried sex, Sue had suffered severe, deep, cutting pains. She was sure that she could never have sex.

"It's so hard," she said. "I spend all my life saying sex is wrong and I won't do it. Now suddenly I'm married; it's okay; and I'm supposed to enjoy it." She knew that God had created her as a sexual being but she found it hard to put into practice what she was created to be.

They had avoided premarital counseling, and we had some catching up to do. Her problem stemmed from misinformation and fear. She had learned from her mother that sex was a disgusting act, forced on women. During sex, her anxiety produced intense vaginal muscle spasms (vaginismus), resulting in unbearable pain.

After several weeks of counseling and a few intimate exercises in their own bedroom, they returned for a follow-up visit. Their honeymoon glow made it clear that divorce was now the last thing on their minds.

Stress and the Heart

One day I (SIM) received an urgent call to see a college student who was "dying from a heart attack." I found him on the floor, gasping for breath and clutching his chest in pain. He sure looked like he was dying but he was in no immediate danger. His heart was healthy, but his spirit was troubled. He was hyperventilating from a panic attack.

We see this problem far more often than real heart attacks. The National Institute of Mental Health reports that one in fourteen adults has suffered panic attacks.[3]

Although stress causes many panic attacks, it triggers many heart attacks as well. On 18 January 1991 the people of Israel suffered an incredible fright. That was the day that Saddam Hussein launched his first Scud-missile attack on Israel. The danger was real, imminent, and uncontrollable. Everyone in Israel was stressed out.

On that day doctors noticed a tremendous increase (58 percent) in the adult death rate. Most of these excess deaths were heart attack victims who arrived at the hospital "DOA" (dead on arrival).[4] During the Gulf War, Scud fear may have killed more people than Scud explosions.

Stress and the Whole Body

Just how important is stress and our emotional response to it? Check out this partial list of diseases caused or worsened by emotional stress. Because much of this information is not included in standard medical texts, we include selected references for doctors, students, or others who wish to do further research.

Disorders of the Digestive System
- Ulcers of the stomach and intestines[5]
- Ulcerative colitis[6]
- Loss of appetite
- Hiccups
- Irritable bowel syndrome
- Swallowing difficulties

Disorders of the Circulatory System
- High blood pressure[7]
- Abnormal heartbeats (premature ventricular contractions, paroxysmal tachycardia, etc.)[8]
- Angina pectoris[9]
- Heart attacks (sudden death and myocardial infarction)[10]
- Strokes[11]

Disorders of the Genito-Urinary Systems
- Lack of menstruation
- Vaginismus
- Frequent or painful urination
- Impotence

- Dysfunctional uterine bleeding[12]
- False pregnancy[13]
- Infertility[14]

Disorders of the Nervous System

- Headaches of most types
- Epilepsy
- Panic attacks
- Tremors
- Suicide

Disorders of Glands

- Thyroid disorders[15]
- Diabetes (types I and II, affecting both the onset and course of disease)[16]
- Chronic pancreatitis[17]

Allergic and Immunologic Disorders

- Chronic fatigue syndrome[18]
- Hives
- Hay fever
- Asthma attacks[19]
- Poor responses to vaccination[20]

Muscle and Joint Disorders

- Low back syndrome
- Neck spasms
- Rheumatoid arthritis[21]
- Myasthenia gravis[22]

Infections

- Common cold[23]
- Infectious mononucleosis[24]
- Chronic tuberculosis[25]
- Strep throat[26]

Inflammatory and Skin Diseases

- Neurodermatitis
- Raynaud's disease[27]
- Systemic lupus erythematosus (SLE)

Nutritional and Drug Disorders

- Anorexia nervosa
- Obesity
- Drug addictions (cocaine, alcohol, nicotine, marijuana, caffeine, etc.)
- Vitamin toxicity

Cancer

- Lung cancer[28]
- Gastric cancer[29]
- Childhood cancers[30]
- Breast cancer[31]
- Cancers of many types[32]

Of course, psychological and spiritual factors rarely act alone in causing or irritating most diseases. Genetics, age, immunizations, nutrition, exercise, and many other factors also play important roles.

In the following chapters we will examine how a healthy spiritual and emotional life generally leads to a healthy physical body. Isaiah told how God had protected his people in the previous centuries:

> You have been
> a strength to the needy in his distress,
> a refuge from the storm,
> a shade from the heat.
>
> Isaiah 25:4

Even during the third millennium:

> In financial stress,
> God can be your strength.
> In relational storms,
> God can be your refuge.
> In the heat of the workplace,
> God can be your shade.

NINETEEN

Public Enemy Number One

He is a killer, responsible for almost one million deaths a year, killing four in ten Americans.

He is a thief, robbing over 260 billion dollars each year.[1]

Mr. Arterio Sclerosis can truthfully be called "Public Enemy Number One."

Modern doctors use many weapons to attack that killer—Mr. Arterio Sclerosis. They arrest him with anticholesterol drugs. They cut him out with bypass surgery. They put the squeeze on him with balloon angioplasty. Still, this cunning criminal outsmarts medicine's greatest minds and torments about fifty-seven million Americans.

Arterio's attacks cause strokes, heart attacks, gangrene, and other fatal conditions. Serious disease and death may occur when he clogs an artery to any major organ.

The Lifesaver Lifestyle

Your lifestyle may be inviting this killer into your life, but you can shut him out by adopting a lifesaver lifestyle. A lifesaver lifestyle includes eating a low-fat diet, losing weight, exercising, quitting smoking, and managing stress.

Low-Fat Diet

Animal fats are a major source of cholesterol and saturated fats. Your body converts saturated fats into cholesterol particles that result in arteriosclerosis.

A nation's cardiac death rate correlates with that nation's meat-fat consumption. Mega–meat fat countries have high death rates. Low–meat fat countries have low coronary death rates.

When you eat animal fats, the next animal you kill may be yourself. Why is cholesterol a killer? Cholesterol deposits in the walls of arteries, forming thick, hard plaques. As these plaques grow, they begin to block off the flow of blood. They may also crack, forming an irregular surface where a clot may form.

The clot blocks blood flow. A part of your heart cries out for oxygen. Crushing chest pain ensues. The heart pump may fail or its electrical system may short-circuit and arrest.

One of four people with heart disease seems healthy until he dies suddenly. The day he discovers that he has heart disease is the day he dies. Waiting to change your diet may be a fatal mistake. You may not get a second chance. After your first warning, you may never eat another meal. *Sixty percent of the victims of fatal heart attacks never reach the hospital.*

You will probably not be surprised to learn that the Bible recorded your modern doctor's advice 3,500 years ago: "Do not eat any of the fat of cattle, sheep or goats" (Lev. 7:22). The Bible specifically forbade eating the fatty portions of the already-lean Palestinian animals.

Amazing! How could primitive Israelites have made this medical advance? Without thousands of researchers. Without billions of dollars. Without modern laboratories. Without checking cholesterol. Without university professors. Without population studies. Without the AMA. Without cholesterol drugs. Without even a significant cardiac death rate. Maybe this healthy directive really did come directly from where Moses said—from God himself.

Losing Weight

Overweight people store animal fat under their own skin. This excess fat accelerates atherosclerosis. If every American were at ideal weight, heart attacks would drop by more than 25 percent and strokes would drop by more than 30 percent.[2]

Dr. W. B. Kannel has said, "Correction of overweight is probably the most important hygienic measure (aside from avoidance of cigarettes) available for the control of cardiovascular disease."[3]

Exercising

Exercise invigorates your heart, reduces your weight, and lowers your cholesterol. Even without any weight loss, exercise reduces your risk for diabetes and heart disease.

Serious exercise was part of God's original plan. God put Adam in the Garden of Eden, "to work it" (Gen. 2:15). In the Ten Commandments, God tells us, "Six days you shall labor and do all your work" (Exod. 20:9). Back then, all work was real exercise: hoeing, planting, harvesting, milling, gathering wood, shepherding, hunting. God didn't say we should merely tolerate vigorous work. No, he encouraged it, blessed it, and even commanded it.

Studies have found that manual laborers, such as farmers and dock workers, suffer fewer heart attacks. In the modern world, however, many other jobs require little physical exertion. If you have one of these sedentary jobs, exercise is critical. Daily exercise will protect you from arteriosclerosis in at least four ways:

- increasing good (HDL) cholesterol blood levels
- increasing blood flow to the heart
- burning up excess fat
- producing a sense of well-being

Discipline in exercise will help you in other areas, such as discipline in diet, discipline in prayer, and disciplining your temper. You will even work more efficiently.

Quitting Smoking

Not convinced? Read chapter seven.
Still need convincing? Read it again.
Not convinced yet? You probably own stock in R. J. Reynolds.

Managing Stress

How can stress on your brain lead to disease in your heart? Stress will raise your blood pressure. One study found that men in high-stress jobs had blood pressures nine points higher than men in low-stress jobs. Three years later the blood pressures of those men who had switched to low-stress jobs dropped an average of four points.[4]

Stress also raises your cholesterol,[5] insulin, and blood sugar levels.[6] These changes accelerate arteriosclerosis. Stress thickens your blood[7] and makes your clotting cells (platelets) stickier.[8] Stress even blocks your body's clot-dissolving enzymes.[9]

If you live overstressed, one day a crack may form in one of your cholesterol plaques. Your sticky platelets will clump there and clot. No blood will get through, and your crushing pain will signal a heart attack. Remember, your first warning may be your last thought.

In real life, stress overload often precedes coronary death. A study was done of 119 apparently healthy men who died suddenly of heart attacks. Over the year prior to their deaths these men ignored the screeching tires of stress. In the quarter before they died their stress level had nearly tripled.[10] Unfortunately they never got a second chance to deal with stress differently; the first warning signal they got was sudden death. Like burned-out tires at Daytona, their hearts simply blew out.

Peace by a River

Stress need not cause blowouts. Consider the stress that my (SIM) wife, Alice, once experienced on a Canadian fishing trip. We arrived at our cabin around 5 P.M. one Saturday. To catch fish for our Sunday meals, my daughter Linda and I rowed up the treacherous Matawan Rapids. Seeing a tree wrapped around a rock like a roll of Play-Doh, I realized that this river demanded respect.

Alice stayed in the cabin to unpack. Then she sat down to await our return. Eight o'clock passed, but no boat came. Nine o'clock, nine-thirty—still no Linda, still no Mack.

Night fishing up the Matawan Rapids was just this side of lunacy, but if Alice had become hysterical, her internal stress would not have brought us any closer. Worse yet, she would have released stress hormones and damaged her own body.

Instead, the Lord reminded her of a verse from a passage we were memorizing that vacation: "I sought the LORD, and he heard me, and delivered me from all my fears" (Ps. 34:4). Alice sought the Lord in prayer, and he truly did deliver her from her fears.

Alice sat alone in the dark, the lantern by her side. Rapids roared. Shadows shivered. Stars sparkled. Alice prayed. At ten o'clock she heard a voice behind her. "Daddy sent me by land. He didn't want to bring me down the rapids in the dark. The fish were slow in biting; but once they started, they bit like a house afire!"

Still more waiting. Ten-thirty—no boat. Only the roaring river answered Alice's calls. She knew that at any moment my hat might float by, but the Lord had given her peace. In her faith, she had power over panic. Power she needed, for it was not until eleven o'clock that the evidence of her faith arrived safely at the dock.

Wherever and whenever Alice and I have experienced fear, we have proven God's promises, and his peace has prevailed.

> In Africa, when we heard midnight drums in the jungle;
>> prayer brought peace.
> In the mid-Atlantic, when a Nazi U-boat stopped our ship
>> during World War II;
>> prayer brought peace.
> In the USA, when our daughter hovered near death from
>> meningitis;
>> prayer brought peace.

Stress will come, and stress will go; but the peace of God can stay for good—

> for the good of your heart,
> and the good of your soul.

TWENTY

The Stress-Free Life

Wouldn't you love to live a stress-free life? The only problem is that the stress-free life doesn't exist. Stress *is* life.[1]

Although people have always experienced stress, the concept of stress did not even exist until the 1930s. We owe the concept of stress to a clumsy, young scientist—Hans Selye. As the story goes, Hans Selye was constantly dropping his lab rats, chasing them around the room, and trapping them in the corner. Worse yet, his experiments weren't working. His rats kept getting ulcers and hormone imbalances.

He wasn't the first scientist to have this problem but he was the genius who figured out what was going on. The stress of being chased and raced was making the rats sick. He borrowed a term from engineering, and the idea of *stress* was born. He went on to found the International Institute of Stress. How would you like to work there?

Many folks, caught in today's rat races, could take a lesson from those rats. Compared to the last generation, we work more hours for a similar paycheck. Our leisure time gets sucked up in carting the kids around, using all our laborsaving devices, and answering the cell phone and e-mail. Meanwhile, modern culture encourages both parents to work full-time, eat low-fat diets, exercise, spend quality time with children, and volunteer for every one of a hundred good causes.

Many of us feel as if we are riding a brakeless tractor trailer hurtling down a steep mountain. We're just struggling to hang on to our sanity for one more minute. We try to do everything, and we end up doing little of permanent significance. No wonder we're stressed out!

Your Stress Test

We have included a stress test (see pages 186–88), so you can see what your level of stress is. Please, take a few minutes now to take the test.

A majority of middle-aged Americans say that they "frequently" experience stress in their daily life.[2] How about you? Has your on-the-edge life put you in quadrant four? Are you heading for a stress attack? If so, there's hope.

In many ways, we decide how much stress to live with. We decide what job to take. We may decide to take a second job. We decide what home to live in. We decide how much or how little time to spend with our children. We decide what to do with our weekends. We may even decide how many children we will have.

Since living on the stressful edge is often a result of our own decisions, we can make different decisions and live a sane-stress life.

My Stress Level

My Lifestyle	almost never	sometimes	usually	almost always
I have trouble getting to sleep or getting up.			X	
My car is a mess.		X		
I sense that my job may not be secure.	X			
I must wait for a check to clear to pay the bills.	X			
I am unable to invest 10 percent of my income for retirement.	X			
I work longer hours than I or my spouse would like.			X	
I wish that I watched less TV.		X		
I have credit card debt.		X		
I weigh more than I want to.		X		
I do not exercise 3 or more times per week.				X
I am not recognized for my contributions at work.	X			
I worry about my or someone else's health.		X		
I am late for appointments.		X		
Arguments at home are not resolved on the same day.		X		
Subtotals	4	7	2	1
	x 1 = 4	x 2 = 14	x 3 = 6	x 4 = 4

Below 28: You are living a low-stress life.
28 and above: You are living a high-stress life.
Find your zone on page 188.

Total Stress Score 28

You Need Stress

Stress is God's plan for your daily life. Does that sound crazy? The Bible says:

> We should rejoice in our difficulties, because we know that:
> suffering leads to perseverance,
> perseverance leads to character,
> and character leads to hope.
> And this kind of hope will not let us down.
>
> Romans 5:3–5

This principle is not just abstract theology. Psychologists now affirm that we all need a certain amount of stress. Dr. Douglas

My Stress Response

Life Event (Choose the highest response that fits you)	0	5	10
Someone cuts me off in traffic.	Poor guy; having a bad day.	Wow. It's dangerous out here.	Crazy driver. #%^%#@
Someone lectures me wrongly in an area of my own expertise.	Maybe he knows something I don't know.	His insecurity is showing. I'll let it pass.	I feel the urge to set him straight.
I hear of a child who died of a drug overdose.	I realize that bad things happen.	We need better drug programs.	I wish the drug pusher were dead.
I am going to have to speak to a large group.	I am ready a week in advance.	I am nervous just before the talk.	I stay awake worrying about it.
I have been waiting an hour for the doctor when someone who came after me checks out.	I assume that there must be a good reason.	I remind the receptionist that I am waiting.	I feel anger and irritation boiling up inside of me.
My mechanic puts on the oil filter incorrectly. The engine is ruined.	Everybody makes mistakes.	I ask for him to pay for the damage.	I want to tell people what a bad job he did.
Layoffs are coming at work, and I sense that my job may be cut.	I try to ignore any negative thoughts.	I consider a new job and prepare a résumé.	I worry or I am furious at management.
My next-door neighbor's house is robbed.	I am thankful that it wasn't me.	I consider a burglar alarm.	I hear imaginary burglars at night.
Dad calls; he says I am making a "big mistake."	He's older, so he must be right.	I consider his advice.	I think, Who asked him?
The weather forecast is wrong and my picnic is ruined.	Great. I get to spend time with my friends.	Maybe I'll use another weather channel next time.	I always blame weathermen for the weather.
Subtotals	x 0 = _3_	x 5 = _5_ 25	x 10 = _2_ 20

Total Response Score _45_

50 and below: *Cool Reactor.* You tend to roll with the punches.
Over 50: *Hot Reactor!* You may not look upset but you tend to respond to stress with a harmful adrenaline rush.
Find your zone on page 188.

Kleiber says, "To be happy, you need to feel a little stressed. It's human nature to thrive when you're challenged. Sometimes you overshoot, try to do too much, and get anxious. Sometimes you don't try hard enough, and get bored. It's a constant adjustment."[3]

Each person has an optimum stress level. Coping with stress develops perseverance and character needed to cope with future stress.

My Stress Zone		
	Low-Stress Life	**High-Stress Life**
Cool Reactor	**I** Great! You are a rare person. Stress is not a problem for you right now. Of course, stressful events will happen to you, but you should be able to roll with the punches.	**II** You have plenty of stress in your life, but you seem to handle it well. Still, anyone can get overloaded, so you may want to lighten your stress load before you start to suffer.
Hot Reactor	**III** You're not stressed out now. But be careful; you tend to overreact to stress. Now is a good time to learn disciplines that will help you keep from overreacting.	**IV** Watch out! You're in the danger zone. Simplify your life. Take a vacation. Learn new ways to handle stress. Stress may be hastening the end of your life.

Understress

The graph on the next page illustrates that understressed people get bored, irritable, and depressed. Maybe this happened to you once when you spent a long weekend vegetating in front of the TV, eating Cheetos. Your muscles felt like soggy potato chips, and your brain like a tub of cheese dip. You were understressed. You had an acute case of blah-itis.

Optimum Stress

In the middle is optimum stress. You have just enough stress to keep you motivated, challenged, and excited about life.

Overstress

For many, the issue is overstress. Remember when you went through a week, working eighteen-hour days, trying to reach a deadline? When you finally realized that you weren't going to make it, your life felt out of control. You were overstressed. You were heading for burnout. If your stress pendulum swings out into overstress, what can you do to avoid burnout?

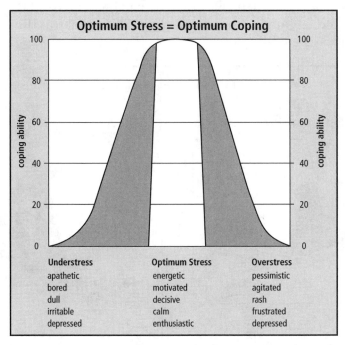

Develop a Sense of Control

Remember the last time you felt really stressed out? Your life felt out of control. No matter how hard you tried, everything seemed out of control. Control is the critical issue in stress. Inner stress is not so much a matter of life's difficulties. *Inner stress is a matter of control.* When you feel you have lost control, you are stressed out.

An experiment illustrates the importance of control. College students were paired and put into separate rooms to solve complex math problems. Identical music was piped into both rooms. Student VC had a volume control, and Student NC had no control. Student NC just listened to whatever volume Student VC selected. Both students experienced identical music volumes. The only difference was that student VC had control and student NC had no volume control.

After the experiment, NC students had higher stress hormone levels and felt much more stressed out. The event was the same. The stress was different.

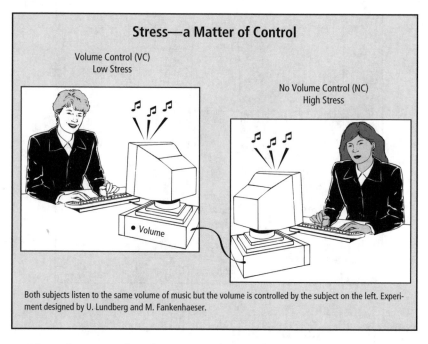

Stress—a Matter of Control

Volume Control (VC)
Low Stress

No Volume Control (NC)
High Stress

Both subjects listen to the same volume of music but the volume is controlled by the subject on the left. Experiment designed by U. Lundberg and M. Fankenhaeser.

If on the stress level test your total stress score was over 35, you are in danger. You have probably lost a sense of control in your life. At times you probably feel like a soccer ball in a playground. Everyone takes a kick at you as he or she goes by, and there is little that you can do about it.

This loss of control is what we perceive as stress. Dr. Robert Eliot, director of the Institute for Stress Medicine in Denver, says, "A lot of overheating comes from a loss of control, which is followed by an invisible physiologic and metabolic struggle. . . . Tell me how much control a person has over what he really wants, and I'll tell you how much stress he has."

On the other hand, people who feel reasonably in control of their lives enjoy work more, expect more raises and promotions, have better relationships, and are generally more satisfied with their lives.[4]

Elderly adults who enter a nursing home often experience great stress and have elevated stress hormones. If social workers teach them how to take control of their situation, their stress levels and stress hormones return to normal.[5] Control is critical.

Is Faith a Loss of Control?

Many psychology professionals are leery of religion. They suspect that when people give control of their lives to God, they lose control. Psychologist Herbert Lefcourt sounds scholarly and authoritative when he says:

> The sense of control, the illusion that one can exercise personal choice, has a definite and positive role in sustaining life. The illusion of freedom is not to be easily dismissed without anticipating undesirable consequences. To submit to however wise a master planner is to surrender an illusion [freedom of choice] that may be the bedrock on which life flourishes.[6]

He is saying that if you put your faith in God, you will lose "the bedrock on which life flourishes." What a frightening thought! If he is right, maybe the government should issue a statement: "Danger. The Surgeon General has determined that faith in God may be harmful to your health."

But Dr. Lefcourt is simply unaware of the scientific evidence. The research on faith and health shows the exact opposite. Study after study has reached the same conclusion: People of faith cope with stress better than people without faith. This is true for stressed-out college students,[7] the elderly,[8] and everyone in between.[9] One research group noted, "Our findings indicate that religion may be a potent coping strategy that facilitates adjustment to the stress of life."[10]

Why is faith such a powerful help in coping with stress? Faith in God allows us to cultivate four disciplines that help us cope with stress:

- Direction
- Balance
- Rest
- A positive attitude

Direction

When a woman of faith encounters a major stress in life, she need not throw up her hands and say, "I have no idea what to do. I'll just sit back and see what God will do." No. The Christian woman can face life as an adventurer with a map. She knows the locations of life's rapids, ravines, and minefields. She sees where the safe havens, fruitful fields, and peaceful waters lie. She may not know everything that will happen but she knows that God will steer her clear of the tar pits of sin. Life is a guided tour with a great destination.

Without God, she had to face life, unsure of its pitfalls and dangers. A little white lie, "Oh no! Now I have to tell another one." A little fudging to the IRS, "I wonder if the statute of limitations is up yet." A little sex outside of marriage, "I hope I don't get caught." Without God, life is a dangerous expedition into the unknown. The stress never stops.

David rejoiced that even in the stresses of life God would give direction:

> The LORD is *my shepherd;* I shall not want.
> He maketh me to *lie down* in green pastures: he *leadeth me beside the still waters.*
> He *restoreth my soul:* he *leadeth me* in the paths of righteousness for his name's sake.
> Yea, though I walk through the valley of the shadow of death, I will *fear no evil:* for *thou art with me.*
>
> Psalm 23:1–4 KJV, emphasis added

In stress, the faithless derail, but those with faith have direction.

Balance

A medical journal has published a diagram showing how we can avoid burnout. It shows that we need to balance three dimensions of our lives—work, play, and worship. Most people live two-dimensional lives, leaving out the critical aspect of worship.

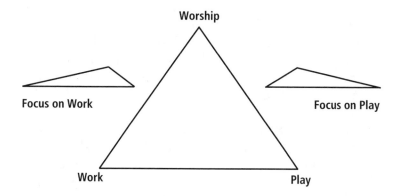

We may avoid worship and overemphasize play or work but we end up with a flat, two-dimensional life. More work or more play will never fill the spiritual dimension. "Lifestyles of the Rich and Famous" may value the workaholic CEO or the playboy millionaire, but their lives are out of balance. Their depressions, divorces, and suicides prove that the two-dimensional life is missing something.

The three-dimensional life of balanced worship, work, and play brings richness and meaning. We have often put in a long day at the office, felt tired, and been tempted to skip small-group Bible study. If we went anyway, as the prayer and fellowship began, we had a sense of meaning and connectedness to God. We felt rejuvenated. If, instead, we had put in a few extra hours at the office, we would have felt even more tired. On other days, we may need a ball game or an evening of table games to balance our life. When we neglect worship, work, or play, our lives are out of balance. Keeping all three in balance refreshes the soul.

Rest

We all need to take regular breaks from life's constant stresses. We often see patients who are paying dearly because they have neglected rest. One study found that 26 percent of men who had suffered heart attacks had been working over seventy hours a week.[11] They had literally worked themselves into the grave.

Jesus knew about stress. At one point he and his disciples were mobbed by "so many people that they couldn't even find time to eat." Jesus said to his disciples, "'Come with me to an out-of-the-way place where we can rest in privacy.' So they got into a boat and sailed to a place of quiet solitude" (Mark 6:31–32).

Every time we visit a lake and feel the boat gliding out into the water, we see the wisdom of Jesus. Nothing shuts out the stresses of daily life like a boat gliding out on the water. Many people would still be alive today if they had followed Jesus' example.

Simple inactivity, however, is not rest. A couch-potato weekend is not refreshing. Twenty hours of TV, three bags of Doritos, and four liters of Coke will not get you ready to attack the next week.

A rest that refreshes must calm the spirit *and* feed the soul. Jesus understood this principle. The Bible reports that, "Jesus often withdrew to quiet places to pray" (Luke 5:16). If Jesus needed worshipful rest, certainly we mere mortals need it too. We need quiet communion with God to feed our souls. God knows our need for rest. That's why he instructs his people to set aside one day in seven as a Sabbath for worshipful rest.

In this solitude, we can find peace during even the most severe stress. Richard J. Foster writes, "In the midst of noise and confusion we are settled into a deep inner silence."[12] In this solitude, God calms our spirit and feeds our soul. This is the rest that refreshes. This is the rest that relieves stress. This is the rest that leaves a person feeling alive and ready to take on any stress the world can dish out.

A Positive Attitude

When it comes to stress, my attitude will determine my altitude. While I (SIM) was catching a minute to write this chapter, my telephone rang. A college nurse was calling, "Doctor McMillen, there's a girl here with her dog. There's a fishhook caught in its ear. I don't know how to take it out, so I am sending her over to your office."

I can remember a time when my response might have broken the phone. More likely, my tirade could have blown a stress fuse, resulting in a pounding headache, a paralyzing stroke, or a fatal heart attack. All this over a simple humanitarian request.

Years ago because of my poor reaction to stress, I nearly died of a bleeding ulcer. In dealing with my ulcer, I became painfully aware of my stomach's reaction to blowing my stress fuses. Much of what I learned from that experience gave birth to the ideas in this book.

We should not blame a boss, coworker, teacher, or spouse for our own ulcers. Our ulcers are really the result of our internal reactions to stress. It is not the stress, but our reaction that is toxic to our body.

Take for example my telephone. Even on my day off, it can be a source of constant interruption. After the first dozen calls, I have a tendency to cringe from these repeated interruptions. If I blow up, I can let a simple ringing telephone ruin my day and cause my ulcer to flare up. I may be tempted to blame the phone, but the phone is not my problem. My problem is my faulty reaction to the calls.

Most of us have been guilty of generating one hundred dollars of adrenaline over a ten-cent incident. In fact getting an answering service that bunches the nonemergency interruptions into a single call is a way for me to take control of my phone stress problem. Instead of the irritation of a constantly ringing phone, the rare ringing of the phone can bring a welcome diversion.

Stress—Fuse Blower or Battery Charger?

On earth, the stress-free life will never arrive. But remember that stress is not the problem. We all need some level of stress to continue living. I can recall many times when I (SIM) had to make a house call when I myself felt ill. Often the mental diversion and the thankful patient relieved my minor aches and pains. If, instead, I had fumed in irritation, neither I nor the patient would have felt any better.

Our *reactions to stress* determine whether stress will *help us* or *hurt us*. The Bible reminds us that our attitudes make the difference: "Everyone who is suffering while doing good, should rest their souls in continuing in doing good" (1 Peter 4:19).

Our reaction to stress is an important key to longer, better living. When we feel stressed out, will we give up or keep going? Will we see it as an irritation or a challenge? Will we blow a fuse or let it charge us up? We hold the key. We can decide whether stress will work for us or against us—whether stress will make us better or bitter.

In life's briar patches, thorny people can make life irritating. If we let irritations nettle our spirits, we may end up with the physical pains of ulcers or heart attacks. If, instead, we learn to understand and even enjoy the idiosyncrasies of life's prickly people, we can rise above the aggravation. A simple attitude adjustment will make their barbs bounce off like thorns on rhino hide.

Paul suffered stress from what he called his "thorn in the flesh." "Three times I pleaded with God to remove it, but God answered, 'My grace is sufficient for you, for in your weakness *you must rely* completely on my power'" (2 Cor. 12:8).

When life's thorns leave us stressed out and we realize that we can't make it alone, we can rely on the perfect power of God.

TWENTY-ONE

The Faith Factor

. . . folklore . . . on the fringes of the research community.

Dr. Jeffrey Levin (1994), on the medical community's attitude toward research linking faith and health

TV networks all miss the story, but it's the world's biggest mega-event. It's bigger than the Super Bowl, World Series, World Cup, and Olympics combined. Even more amazing, it happens every week. It's church.

Maybe you attended church last Sunday. If so, did you know that you were nourishing both your soul and body? Faith is strong medicine. It can prevent and even cure many diseases. When doctors first hear this, many frown in doubt. "Give me a break," they say. "Religion is superstition. Medicine is science."

Doctors may recall a dying patient, who claimed the miracle cure that never came. They may remember a schizophrenic, who shouted that he was the Messiah. Faith may make death more tolerable, but doctors doubt that it makes life any healthier.

Point	**Counterpoint**
Destroy yourself physically and mentally; and insist that all true believers do likewise as an expression of unity.	Your body is a temple of the Holy Spirit. . . . Therefore honor God with your body.

Robert Hunter,
*The Ten Commandments
of Rock and Roll*

God, *The Bible*

One Man's Story

Skeptics are nothing new. One hundred years ago, in the coal-mining town of Barnesborough, Pennsylvania, the town doctor was a hard-core skeptic. Once he had been a church deacon and a community leader—a vigorous, healthy man. Then, no one knows exactly what happened, but he changed. He quit church and constantly bashed religion. He physically abused his wife and children. Anger filled his heart, and health drained from his body.

The doctor had a son he neglected. He didn't even bother to name the boy, so folks just called him, "Guy" or "Hey you." At the age of eight, the boy named himself—Sim Isocrates. Sim spent Friday nights in saloons, where he bummed pretzels from drunken coal miners. More than once, he watched bloody brawls spill out into the street. The boy seemed destined for despair, drunkenness, and disease.

Then, Sim's older sister Oneida enraged her father by becoming a born-again Christian. When she left home to enter church work, he exploded, "Go! But if you die up there, let them bury you up there. I don't ever want to see your face again."

Oneida left.

The doctor was only fifty-five, but he became deathly ill. Bedridden and bankrupt, he had to sell his house and move to

Oneida's home. There, his once-disowned daughter tenderly nursed him on his deathbed. He rarely thanked her, yet she radiated a strange joy and love.

Sim longed to know the source of her love. One night he accepted Jesus and found it. Suddenly his soul was bathed in an overwhelming love, the love of his heavenly Father—a Father who would never abuse or leave him. Sim's life was transformed.

Supporting himself, he graduated from college and medical school. He traveled to Africa, built a mission hospital, and discovered a cure for noma—a fatal children's disease.

His father had died at fifty-five, but that abused orphan lived well into his nineties. His name was Dr. S. I. McMillen; and you are now reading the latest revision of his book.

Dr. McMillen never took personal credit for his health or accomplishments. Frequently, he would say, "I hate to think where I would be without Jesus." His father chose a godless path and it led to disease and early death. Dr. McMillen traveled the path of faith, and it led to health and long life.

And now you know the rest of this story.

Faith Makes Fit

Still, skeptics might argue that Dr. McMillen's faith did not make his life long and healthy. Maybe he was just lucky.

Remember back in 1863, skeptics mocked Dr. Semmelweis's idea for handwashing. In 1963 similar skeptics scoffed at the new book *None of These Diseases.* A famous surgeon called it "shallow" and "naive." Could faith really produce health? Could church visits really reduce hospital visits? Could prayer really replace pills? Back then, skeptics had a point, for few studies had yet looked at these questions.

Since then, however, hundreds of studies have examined the relationship of faith and health. Eighty to ninety percent of these studies have reached the same conclusion: Faith makes fit, and doubt makes sick.

Religiosity is in many respects equivalent to irrational thinking and emotional disturbance. . . . The less religious they are, the more emotionally healthy they will be.

Albert Ellis, psychologist

There has not been one [of my patients] whose problem in the last resort was not that of finding a religious outlook on life. . . . None of them has been really healed who did not regain his religious outlook.

Carl Jung, founder of analytical psychology

In 1995 more than one thousand health professionals attended a Harvard Medical School conference on the subject of faith and health. *Internal Medicine News* headlined the meeting, "Experts Call Spirituality an Untapped Therapy."[1] Weekly church attendance, daily Bible reading, and a constant attitude of prayer are great medicines for mind, body, and soul.

One study reviewed at this conference found that weekly churchgoers in Maryland were less likely to die from:

- heart attacks (50 percent reduction)
- emphysema (56 percent reduction)
- cirrhosis (74 percent reduction)
- and suicide (53 percent reduction)[2]

Devout churchgoers have been found to fare better than the irreligious as:

- heart attack patients at Dartmouth University[3]
- hip fracture patients at Northwestern University[4]
- and geriatric patients seen at Yale University[5]

Medicine and religion are the twin traditions of healing. They grew up together and became separated in early childhood. As we approach the third millennium, maybe they can come back together.

Dale Matthews, M.D., Georgetown University

Faith has been found to be beneficial in the prevention and treatment of many conditions. Even when studies factor out the effects of smoking and drinking, the health benefits of faith usually remain.

Of course not every devout believer experiences perfect health all the time. Some may suffer trials of cancer, heart attacks, and other illnesses. But in general, believers are healthier than nonbelievers.

Jesus himself expected faith to heal both body and soul. He even used the same Greek verb (*sōzō)* for healing the body and saving the soul. He told blind Bartimaeus, "Your faith has *healed* [*sōzō*] you" (Mark 10:52). After forgiving a woman's sins, he spoke the identical phrase, "Your faith has *saved* [*sōzō*] you." (Luke 7:50).[6]

Atheist Karl Marx ridiculed religion as "the opium of the masses"; but as usual, Marx missed the mark. Faith may be strong medicine, but it is no numbing narcotic. Faith is an essential factor for fortifying the health of both body and soul.

New Age Health

Today many people reject formal religion but they are still spiritually curious. They shop for religion like they shop for a car. They don't want a boring Buick; they want a faith Ferrari. They will choose the color, the interior, and all the extras. They may select an idol of Buddha, a mantra from Krishna, a teaching from Jesus, a crystal from a Navaho, and any other spiritual option that may suit their fancy.

New Age religion, however, is nothing new. It's as old as the Old Testament. Jeremiah lamented that "each one chooses his own path" (Jer. 8:6). He scolded Israel for mixing temple worship with household idols and for mixing pious prayer with mountaintop occultism.

Throughout the twentieth century, people were fascinated with mix-and-match religions. One writer describes 1910 London: "There was a widespread taste among intellectuals for esoteric religions and cults . . . psychic phenomena and sexual freedom. . . . Many of the cults were ascribed to the East, but the leaders . . . often [called themselves] Christians."[7]

Today's New Agers often add health awareness to the mix. They tout herbs, vitamins, and cosmic health forces. New Ager Beverly Barré says, "Taking care of yourself is a religion."[8]

But does New Age religion really lead to better health? No. Studies indicate that New Age beliefs may actually harm your health. Spiritual growth requires change, but New Agers invent a religion to make themselves feel good, not to change themselves. If they have unhealthy habits of envy, anger, or pride, their new religion simply justifies their vices. New Agers mold their faith to fit their lifestyles, but biblical Christians must mold their lifestyles to fit their faith. That means big changes—repentance, regeneration, and holiness.

Duke psychiatrist Redford Williams comments, "[People] who find religion useful but selectively shape their creed to fit their other interests, tend to be less mentally healthy."[9]

A Healthy Faith

What sort of faith constitutes the faith factor? One expert, Dr. Jeffrey Levin, has noted a reoccurring theme in the medical research. Avoiding traditional faith appears to be a risk factor for poor health. Those who benefit most from faith are, in his words, members of the more "behaviorally strict religions or denominations"[10]—what the press tends to lump together as "fundamentalists." Science seems to have rediscovered what the psalmist noted thousands of years ago, "The fear of the LORD prolongs life" (Prov. 10:27).

"The Faith That Heals"
Title of a 1910 paper by Sir William Osler, considered by many to be the greatest American physician ever

---

So should you attend a traditional church as a life-extension program? Probably not. You won't benefit from merely visiting a health food store (or church). Merely buying vitamins (or tithing) won't help. Watching other folks take vitamins (or worship) won't help. Vitamins and faith won't do you any good unless you use them yourself. One secular doctor goes so far as recommending that you "become a truly practicing [church] member, practicing whatever is preached with all your heart."[11]

Why does faith produce health? Much of the benefit comes from the powerful chemical and hormonal changes that faith produces in our bodies.

What if you wake up in the morning and say, "I'm a cosmic evolutionary accident. Everyone around me is just an accident. My whole life is just a series of accidents. I wonder what accident will happen to me today." Your negative outlook will produce fear and doubt in your mind. That fear and doubt will release harmful chemicals from every organ in your body. Those chemicals will wear and tear on your body. When you go to bed that night, you will feel like one day has aged you one decade.

But what if you wake up and say, "Wow! God, thanks for making me your wonderful creation. What blessings will you shower on me today? How will you use me today to bless others?" Then you start your day with a half hour of Scripture reading and prayer.

That's utilizing the faith factor. Your attitude of faith will invigorate your mind and energize your immune system. Every cell in your body will be bathed in soothing chemicals. Your white cells will scarf up invading bacteria. Your blood pressure will smoothly waltz through the day. Your brain cells will crackle with lightning-quick decisions. You will crawl into bed feeling a day younger and you will jump out of bed with the same energy tomorrow.

Do you want to go through life as a cosmic accident, in fear of some health-ruining calamity? Or do you want to go through life as God's creation, with God's creative energy invigorating your body and soul?

To exclude God from psychiatric consultation is a form of malpractice. Spirituality is wonder, joy, and shouldn't be left in the clinical closet.
Arthur Kornhaber, psychiatrist, 1992

Dr. Benjamin Rush, the father of American psychiatry, stated that faith "is as essential to the mind of man as air is to respiration."[12]

For your health, you may attend to the exercise factor, the nutrition factor, and even the stress factor. But maybe today you need to consider and apply the antidote to the lethal toxins of doubt, despair, and discouragement. Maybe today it's time to apply the faith factor to your life.

TWENTY-TWO

Danger—Anger

> Getting [habitually] angry is like taking a small dose of some slow-acting poison—arsenic, for example—every day of your life.
>
> Dr. Redford Williams and Dr. Virginia Williams, *Anger Kills*

DANGER: ANGER OVERLOAD. Too bad our emotional dashboards aren't wired to flash this alarm. Instead, we may suffer other anger overload signs—migraines, neck spasms, ulcers, among others.

Feeling angry is as normal as feeling hungry or feeling tired. But anger overload happens when we make a habit of responding to even minor irritations with an anger response. This ingrained anger habit is called hostility.

Anger places every cell in your entire body on red alert. Your stomach churns out acid. Your skin hairs stand upright. Your adrenal glands pour out adrenaline and steroids. Your pupils dilate. Your blood pressure shoots up. Your pulse races. You are ready to run or gun.

What a great response—if someone has just broken into your house! But what if you have an anger habit? What if your toddler has just spilled your coffee? What if a driver cuts you off in traffic? What if a shopper takes eleven items into the ten-item express line? If these minor irritations make you blow your stack, you probably have an anger habit. Your emotional dashboard may be on non-stop anger overload. Years of living on the angry edge can kill you.

One day a man came into my (SIM) office with his young son. The father announced, "I only came to get some more pills for my wife's colitis."

Instantly his son quipped, "Who was Ma colliding with this time?"

We laughed, but indeed her cramping pains of "colitis" (i.e., irritable bowel syndrome or IBS) probably did result from her chronic anger. Millions suffer IBS—the most common gastrointestinal disease. Their emotional centers are hardwired to their intestines. Fits of anger can lead to gut-wrenching nausea, vomiting, cramping, constipation, and diarrhea.

Long-Term Anger—Short-Term Life

Worse than intestinal upset, hostility can kill you. Famous physiologist Dr. John Hunter knew the danger; for he had both a bad heart and a bad temper. He once said, "The first scoundrel that gets me angry will kill me."

One day Dr. Hunter was attending a medical lecture. While the speaker spouted off some ridiculous ideas, Dr. Hunter fidgeted angrily. Finally, he could take it no longer. He jumped to his feet and chewed out the speaker. But Dr. Hunter didn't finish his anger attack, for he suddenly fell dead of a heart attack.

His colleague may have been guilty of bad science but he was not the "scoundrel" who killed Dr. Hunter. Dr. Hunter had overloaded his own anger circuits and blown his own fuse.

Dr. Hunter had a chronic anger problem, but what about you and me? Do we have hostility problems? Maybe. About one person in five has a serious form of "grudgitis." Many of the rest of us have milder cases.

For most of the twentieth century, medical experts did not consider hostility to be a major health risk. They knew the dangers of high cholesterol, high blood sugar, and high blood pressure; but few worried about high hostility.

Hostility shortens the life.
Ecclesiasticus 30:24

Finally, in 1981 scientists at the University of North Carolina found convincing evidence that grudgitis is a major killer. Twenty years earlier researchers had tested hostility levels in 255 medical students. Over the following years, the researchers watched the doctors with high hostility die like raging bulls in a bull ring. By middle age, *13 percent of the high-hostility men had died.* In contrast, *only 2 percent with low hostility had died.* The men with grudgitis had more hypertension and five times more heart attacks. Chronic anger had raised their blood pressure and clogged their coronary arteries. Long-term anger makes for a short-term life.

Aging and Raging

I (DES) first met Jack after he had injured his back at work. I diagnosed a simple back strain, but Jack didn't get better. We tried muscle relaxers, pain medicines, physical therapy, ultrasound treatments, a back brace, injecting trigger points. Nothing helped.

A specialist turned his chart into alphabet soup (CAT scan, MRI, EMG, CBC, RF, ESR, ANA), but still nothing turned up positive. Then I scheduled an extended visit to try to dig up the root cause of his pain. "So Jack," I said. "Tell me again; what caused your injury?"

"You know," said Jack. "I was lifting a bag at work."

"But Jack," I said. "You've lifted thousands of bags. You're a strong man. Why did you get hurt *this time?*"

Almost like a Hollywood special effect, Jack morphed from a golden retriever to a pit bull. "It's all Margola's fault," Jack snarled. "He expects me to load one hundred bags an hour. It's impossible. No wonder I got hurt. He thought I would just sit there and take it but I showed him. No one can take that kind

---

of abuse, not even me. He has no idea what it takes to do my job. Now look what he's got, a worker that's costing him big bucks on disability."

He that adds no fuel to the fire has already put it out.
In the same way, he that does not feed his anger at first
nor blow on the fire himself, has prevented
and extinguished it.

Plutarch, c. A.D. 100

Poor Jack was so angry that he even saw his disability as a way to get back at his boss.

"You seem angry," I said.

"You got that right. I used to worry about it but now I just let it out. If something's buggin' me, I'll let you know it. I don't bottle it up. I don't want to get some sort of disease."

But Jack's approach didn't seem to be working. Like an over-wound spring, his chronic anger was twisting his back into constant spasms. One year and four jobs later, Jack's pit bull face returned at any mention of his old boss.

The Ventilation Myth

Jack's anger theory is widespread: "Get the anger out. Then you will feel better." The idea goes back to Freud, who pictured people as emotional teapots. Unventilated rage, like trapped steam, built up emotional pressure. If you didn't release the anger, it could explode as a neurosis or mental meltdown. Freud would have agreed with Jack: "Pop your lid; blow off the steam."

Popular View

If rage can come out, it can spend itself and be done with. . . . It's not the hatred expressed that's the problem; it's the hatred swallowed.

John Bradshaw

Biblical View

Make a break with old habits — anger, rage, meanness, slanderous gossip and spiteful talk.

Colossians 3:8

Before Freud, civilized people recognized the powerful destructive forces in unrestrained anger. The ancient philosophers had encouraged people to avoid aggression and to use their brainpower to gain self-control. Freud changed all that. He said it was healthy, even necessary, to explode.

Freud's ventilation myth remains firmly embedded in popular culture. Pop psychologists still recommend ventilation or "get-the-anger-out" therapy: screaming, yelling, kicking, punching, howling, or any other outburst you won't get arrested for.

Many studies, however, suggest that ventilation doesn't work.[1] One study evaluated one hundred engineers, recently laid off when their aerospace company downsized. The engineers were angry and they had a right to be angry. They had quit other jobs, uprooted their families, and moved to San Diego. They had been promised three-year jobs; but after only one year, they had all been fired.

Researchers divided them into three groups. Researchers spent time with each group, asking them questions:

- Group 1: questions probing for hostility toward the company (for example, "How has the company been unfair to you?")
- Group 2: questions probing for hostility toward supervisors (for example, "How could your supervisor have prevented your layoff?")
- Group 3: probing with neutral questions (for example, "What is your opinion of the technical library?")

Men who had discussed the wrongs done them became *much angrier after ventilating* their anger. On the other hand, those in group 3, who had *not ventilated* anger, were *less angry*.[2]

People hurt by divorce may also fall prey to the ventilation trap. Some have recorded a mental tape of their ex-spouse's every sin. They constantly replay that tape for anyone who will listen. But the more they rehearse their anger, the more it intensifies. Ten years later, the tape is still running. Everyone they know wants to grab them by the shoulders and shout, "Let it go!"

"Letting off steam" may be a great picture, but you and I aren't teapots. Study after study has reached the same conclusion: *Hashing and rehashing anger does not release anger; it rekindles it, reinforces it, and reaffirms it.*

> When you allow a child to scream, kick, hit or smash objects . . . you are not reducing the child's anger. You are increasing his aggressiveness. You are teaching a cathartic habit.
>
> Carol Tavris, *Anger: The Misunderstood Emotion*

The Bible says, "A fool ventilates anger, but a wise person stays in control" (Prov. 29:11). God's Word—not Freud's—has stood the test of time.

TWENTY-THREE

The High Cost of Getting Even

"Wow! 218 over 122," I (DES) said. "That's your record, Janice. Did you forget your blood pressure pills?"

"Oh no, Doc. I took my pills, but you should have seen what happened out in your parking lot. A kid backed right into my new Cadillac. I let him have it. I'm surprised you didn't hear me in here."

What a shame! That educated, professional woman was risking a stroke, just for the satisfaction of blowing her top. Her car was still as dented as before her explosion.

Why do we jokingly accept our angry outbursts with excuses like, "That's just the way I am"? Why do we humans allow acid anger to fume and corrode mind, body, and soul?

Jesus gave a simple answer. It's a spiritual problem.

One day, a Samaritan town put up a "no vacancy" sign for Jesus and his disciples. They had a policy, "No Jews allowed"; and they were going to enforce it.

James and John blew up. What right did those racist bigots have to refuse the Messiah a hotel room? They wanted to nuke the town with a lightning bolt from heaven. Jesus rebuked them, "You don't realize what *spirit* has taken control of you" (Luke 9:55).

Peter also struggled with his vengeful spirit. At the arrest of Jesus, Peter rushed to cut off his enemy's head. Fortunately he missed; but he wasn't the last vengeful church leader to try to behead an opponent.

"No more of this," Jesus rebuked Peter. "Put your sword away. Don't you realize that anyone who lives by the sword will die by the sword?" (Luke 22:51; Matt. 26:52).

Who is in control of your life—a spirit of revenge or the Holy Spirit?

Give someone
a piece of your mind,
and you give away
your peace of mind.

Soul Slavery

A few years ago, I (SIM) treated a college student—we'll call him Pierre—who suffered constant stomach pains. I saw him many times and ordered many tests, but every one came back normal. The newest medicines gave him only partial relief. A specialist found no specific problem.

After observing his tense personality for several months, I suggested that emotional stress might lie at the root of his problem. He scoffed at the idea.

Pierre was a puzzle until another student told me of a tirade he had heard Pierre deliver. For over an hour, Pierre had stood rigid, excoriating his enemies for swindling his grandfather decades ago. Sweat poured down his red face, but he didn't stop once to wipe his forehead. When he was done, his voice was hoarse and his shirt soaked.

At his next appointment, I asked Pierre about this incident. I used pictures to show him how emotional stress could overstimulate stomach acid secretion. He wasn't interested. All he wanted to know was the name of the "jerk" who had told me the story.

His abdominal pain became so severe that he failed the next semester and left college. He had given up both his health and education. Still, he clung to his acid resentments, as if they were a priceless heirloom. Pierre never realized that the person his hatred harmed the most was himself.

This principle applies even to physical altercations. We have treated scores of young men for fist fight injuries—rarely for broken jaws, but often for broken knuckles. Doctors even call a specific hand fracture the "boxer's fracture." The person throwing the punch is the most likely person to get hurt.

The moment I begin to hate a man, I become his slave. He controls my thoughts. He controls my feelings. He even controls my dreams. Stress hormones constantly surge through my bloodstream and wear down my body. My work becomes drudgery. I tire easily. My windowed office seems like a cell in Alcatraz. Even while sailing the Chesapeake Bay, resentment ruins my relaxation. The spinnaker may be billowing in the breeze, but I might as well be a seasick galley slave.

The one I hate hounds me wherever I go. I can't escape his mental tyranny. The waiter at the seaside restaurant may be serving up a blackened swordfish or a chocolate mousse, but I feel like a dungeon prisoner eating stale bread and musty water. My teeth chew the food, but the one I hate has stolen my pleasure. King Solomon must have had a similar experience, for he wrote: "Better a simple salad with love, than a sumptuous feast with hostility" (Prov. 15:17).

The man I hate may be soundly snoring many miles from my bedroom; but more cruel than any slave driver, he whips my thoughts into a frenzy. My Perfect Sleeper mattress becomes a rack of torture. I am, indeed, a slave to everyone I hate.

> I will not let any man reduce my soul
> to the level of hatred.
>
> Booker T. Washington

Transformation

Despite three years with Jesus, the disciples had remained furious fishermen. Jesus even nicknamed the short-fused James and John the "Sons of Thunder." But then they experienced the power of the Holy Spirit. The Spirit transformed these angry anglers into the greatest teachers of the greatest love of the greatest man who ever lived.

Peter and James died as martyrs without a trace of bitterness. John, the same man who once wished his enemies barbecued by lightning, later wrote: "Anyone who does not LOVE is really dead. Anyone who hates his brother is a murderer, and you are fully aware that a saved murderer is a contradiction in terms" (1 John 3:14–15).

The seventh chapter of Acts records how Stephen "being full of the Holy Spirit" reacted, while being murdered in a hailstorm of rocks. Bones broken and flesh shredded, Stephen showed no spirit of revenge. Just before sinking into a coma, he gasped the same words Jesus used on the cross, "Lord, don't hold this sin against them" (Acts 7:60). How many of us would use our last breath to pray for the spiritual welfare of our own murderers?

We might answer that question by taking a little personal inventory. Yesterday, how did I respond when someone irritated me? At my work, did I throw back the stones or insults? In my car, did I call down fire or curses on other drivers? In conversations, did I cut off heads or reputations? Or was the Holy Spirit of forgiveness in control? Did I try to understand their feelings? Was I gentle with their souls? That was the example of Jesus.

Among our patients, we have seen scores of angry men and women transformed by the power of the Spirit. Dr. Redford Williams, director of behavioral research at Duke University, has also seen these transformed people:

[I have] frequently encountered patients, especially men in their late twenties and early thirties, who say that their religious conversion transformed their lives. Before embracing a religion, they overindulged in alcohol, drove cars recklessly, or abused their wives and children. After conversion, particularly if they remained active participants in their religion, they cut back on alcohol, controlled their pursuit of thrills, and were kinder, gentler husbands and fathers.

We have no hesitation in advising that for many people, becoming more religious can be a very effective antidote for hostility and anger.[1]

What an observation! Even a doctor who has no particular point to prove has been astounded by this transformation. He may credit "religion," instead of the power of God. He may not understand it, but his words are testimony to God's miracle-working power. God is still in the business of changing lives, and no one is too far gone for him to help.

A Killer Transformed

There once lived an angry racist. He joined lynch mobs for sport. He dedicated his life to hunting down and murdering his enemies. But then something radical happened to this hostile human. God transformed him into what he called a "new creation." He went on to write classic books on love and forgiveness. You know him as the apostle Paul.

Paul was highly educated in Greek philosophy, so one might expect his view to mirror Aristotle who wrote, "When a man retaliates there is an end of the matter. The pain of resentment is replaced by the pleasure of obtaining revenge, and so his anger ceases."[2]

But Paul's writings on anger show no hint of his Greek education. Instead he wrote:

Kill off every part of you that belongs to your earthly nature. . . .
Give up your old habits—anger, rage, meanness, slanderous gos-

sip and spiteful talk. . . . Instead . . . form new habits: compassion, kindness, humility, meekness and patience. Be patient with the faults of others, and forgive whoever wrongs you, just as the Lord forgave you.

In summary, make a habit of LOVE.

Colossians 3:5, 7–10, 12–14

As with Paul, the Spirit's transformation is not some magical, once-for-a-lifetime event. It is a daily struggle. As Paul said, it is a matter of unlearning the old habits of hostility and learning to "make a habit of LOVE."

Every day Paul had to crucify his "right" to get even. Every day he had to allow Christ to drive nails into every vengeful bone in his body. The secret to life is not killing yourself by hating your enemies, but killing your self-centeredness by loving your enemies.

"None of these [revenge-produced] diseases"—this can be God's gift to you.

24

Mind over Madder

Nurse your grudge,
  poison your body.
Poison your grudge,
  nurse your body.

On entering the exam room, I (DES) noticed that Steve—a twenty-five-year-old engineer—was obviously upset.

"What's the matter, Steve?" I asked.

"I need Prozac," he said. "I can't sleep . . . My stomach's upset . . . I'm getting headaches . . . I can't take it any longer . . . It's all my mother's fault; she's trying to run my whole life . . ."

"Steve," I said, "you have been living with your mother for twenty-five years now. Has something changed recently?"

Out poured the rest of the story. An old high school flame had called out of the blue the previous week. The next morning, he woke up in her bed.

Since then, Teri had been phoning him several times every day. She wanted to know what clothes he was going to wear, what time he would get up, what he had for dinner, and so on. "I think I love her," he said, "but she won't leave me alone. Even worse, Mom hates her."

"Steve," I said, "are you afraid that Teri wants to run your life just like your mother does?"

He broke down and cried. "Yes," he said, "I can't stand it. Sometimes, I'm afraid that I might get violent . . ."

We spent the next twenty minutes getting to understand his anger and developing an anger action plan. At the end of his appointment, I asked, "Do you still think you need Prozac?"

"No," he said. "I'm okay. I know what I need to do."

Since he was an engineer, he was used to designing and doing experiments. He actually went right out and executed his anger action plan.

When I saw him several months later, he had taken control of his anger problem. He had said good-bye to Teri, obtained an unlisted phone number, and set firm boundaries with his mother. His fear of Teri's domination was gone, and his frustration with his mother was now manageable.

The Anger Alarm

Anger is dangerous but it's not always bad in itself. Anger is like a smoke alarm, telling you that an emotional fire needs to be extinguished. Steve's anger indicated that he had a problem, so he went out and fixed the problem. Then his anger disappeared.

The Bible says, "Be angry, but do not sin" (Eph. 4:26). What does that mean? The next sentence makes it clear: "Don't let the sun go down on your anger." In other words, it's okay to feel angry, but use your anger as an alarm, warning you to take care of a problem immediately. Few of us would ignore a blaring smoke detector, so why ignore our blaring anger detectors?

For Steve, taking Prozac would have been like wearing earplugs to tune out a smoke alarm. On Prozac the anger alarm might not have bothered him much, but his problem would still have been burning out of control.

Use Your Massive Brain

What should you do when you feel angry? Psychologist Dr. Neil Clark Warren suggests:

> Put your massive brain in gear. You have a massive brain capable of tremendous feats. But if you are like most people, you regularly use only a fraction of your brain's potential power. . . . When it comes to anger expression, the challenge you face is to learn to use your rational capacity effectively.[1]

Putting out the flames of anger is harder than putting out a kitchen fire but it is even more important. Ignoring a kitchen fire can burn down your house; ignoring your anger may incinerate your health or relationships.

Next time you get angry, put your massive brain in gear and ask yourself these six questions:

1. Why Did He Do That?

Try to put yourself in the other person's situation. Maybe she was rushed and didn't mean to ignore you. Maybe he had your best interest at heart, for you needed to hear those painful words. Whatever the reason, sitting down and reasoning with yourself may actually put the anger fire out before you go any further.

Research has found this approach to work. In one study, a child bullied some third graders. Researchers then encouraged:

- some children to "talk out" their anger
- some to "blow off steam" by getting revenge

- some to understand the bully by telling them he was sick or tired

Talking about their anger left the children angrier and getting revenge made them more vengeful. But a reasonable explanation for the bully's behavior cooled them down. When they viewed the bully's behavior as forgivable, their anger abated.[2]

Proverbs 19:11 says: "A wise person is slow to anger; to his credit, he will overlook an offense." This is still good advice.

2. Is It Worth the Effort?

"Doctor, I hope you (SIM) can help us. We've driven a long way to see you. We should be enjoying our retirement but for the last few months we haven't been able to sleep, even if we take sleeping pills. I'm getting stomach pains, and Ellen is getting chest pains. The doctors can't figure out what is wrong."

After a thorough medical examination, their problems still left me puzzled. Then Ellen pulled out a letter. "Doctor, you may think I am foolish, but our troubles seemed to start right after we got this letter."

> Dear George,
>   I understand that you are selling some eggs to Harry. You know that I have invested considerable money in the chicken business and can supply more eggs to the people of this little hamlet than they can eat. You ought to know that my business is hurt by your dabbling around with a few hens and selling eggs to Harry. I think you ought to stop.
>
>   Manning Caspar

Ellen was dabbing tears from her cheeks. "We had a right to sell those eggs to Harry," she said. "He preferred our brown eggs to his white ones. But now Manning won't even talk to us. It just makes me so angry. We've never had an experience like this. I think our whole problem stems from eggs—just eggs."

She suggested that they go home and give up their small egg business. It seemed worth a try. They did have a right to sell the eggs, but the few dollars of sales hardly seemed worth hundreds of dollars of medical expenses. Standing up for their rights would only cost them more money and more hassle.

They dropped the egg business and rapidly recovered.

Solomon must have seen this happen many times, for he wrote, "Starting a quarrel is like breaking a dam. So drop the matter before a fight ensues" (Prov. 17:14). If your concern isn't worth the hassle, follow Solomon's advice, "drop the matter."

3. What Are My Primary Emotions?

Aggravations produce sparks of *hurt, fear,* or *frustration* (primary emotions). When these sparks produce enough heat, your emotions ignite and you feel anger (a secondary emotion).

Anger is a nonspecific reaction. Like flames from a fire, it tells you *something* is wrong. But anger can't tell you *what* is wrong, any more than flames tell you what started the fire. To find out what started your fires of anger, you have to investigate.

Ask yourself, "Why am I angry? Am I *hurt, afraid,* or *frustrated?*"

When I first asked Steve what was making him so angry, he said that Teri and his mother were wrong and it made him angry. As long as Steve focused on his anger, he would remain angry. Instead, he had to step back and evaluate his primary emotions. Steve felt *frustrated* with his overbearing mother. Second, he *feared* that Toni would also dominate his life. His frustrations and fears had continued, so his emotional center was burning with anger. If he dealt with his *frustrations* and *fears,* his anger would run out of fuel and burn out.

Anger is a *you* emotion; *"you* make me *angry."* Fear (or *hurt* and *frustration*) are *I* emotions; *"I* am *afraid."* The moment you focus on your feelings instead of the wrong done by someone else, the fire of anger begins to cool. Just evaluating his primary emotions helped Steve cool down. When he understood his anger, he was ready to move toward an anger action plan.

4. What Are My Goals?

Next, decide what it will take to ease your fear, hurt, or frustration.

Steve was an adult. It was okay for him to want to be free of his mother's domination. Many times Steve had told his mother of his wishes, but she had completely ignored him. She would say, "I am your mother. I have a right to be involved in your life." This was true, to a point, but she had failed to transition from a relationship that had been appropriate when Steve had been in junior high. They needed to relate as adult to adult, not parent to child.

His relationship with Teri was not love, it was harassment. He had to end the relationship.

Now, he knew his ultimate goals:

- To reduce his *frustration,* he had to lay down boundaries with his mother and then stick to them.
- To reduce his *fear,* he needed to end his relationship with Teri.

Before you enter an anger action plan, decide on your goals. Then you are ready to proceed.

5. Am I Cooled Off?

If you are still at the boiling point, *stop!* You are not ready to go forward. Take a time-out. Thomas Jefferson said, "When angry, count ten before you speak. If very angry, an hundred." Jefferson was right. Moving ahead in anger will only pour gasoline on the bonfire. Your anger will get hotter, and you might even get burned. Count to a million if you must, but wait until your temper has cooled off before proceeding with your anger action plan.

6. Do I Need an Extra Massive Brain?

Sometimes we are so emotionally distressed that we can't see the situation clearly. In these cases, your emotions may overwhelm your own massive brain. You may need the help of another massive brain—a pastor or therapist.

This happened to me (DES) when my extended family allowed a family feud to fester. Nasty letters were being written. Some relatives wouldn't talk to other relatives. Every time someone tried to fix the problem, it only got worse.

This went on for years, until we chose a wise counselor. Within three months, we had uncovered a host of misunderstandings, agreed on our goals, and developed an anger action plan. Everyone agreed and stuck to it. Years later, the plan is still keeping the family at peace.

If you are involved in a long-term feud, it may be foolish to try to handle the matter yourself. Proverbs 12:15 suggests, "A fool is cocksure of his own plans, but a wise person seeks advice." Before you go on, think about it. Maybe only a fool would try to solve this problem without professional help.

An Anger Action Plan

In other situations, your own massive brain is more than enough to help you work out the problem. You may have heard Doug Lewellen of the People's Court say, "If you have a problem with [such and such], don't take matters into your own hands. You take them to court." That may be the modern American way, but Jesus had a different idea. He said that if you had a disagreement with someone, don't take him to court. Instead, "Settle the matter as soon as you can" (Matt. 5:25). The biblical plan is much more likely to work, and it's much easier on the checkbook.

You may need to find a good time to sit down and talk with the person. Remember, don't just ventilate your anger. Instead, state what happened and say how it made you feel. Make a statement like, "When you _____, *I felt [hurt, afraid,* or *frustrated]."* Let the person respond, and see if you can work it out. If not, don't give up. See if a pastor or counselor can help.

Jesus said that if you have something against someone, then you should go to that person and make things right (Matt. 18:15). What pain we could all avoid, if we all followed Jesus' advice!

For further reading on this subject, we suggest *Make Anger Your Ally* by Neil Clark Warren published by Focus on the Family in 1993.

PART 5

SPIRITUAL
WHOLENESS

TWENTY-FIVE

Tears: Eternity's Contact Lenses

I am sure it is never sadness—a proper straight response to loss—that does people harm, but all the other things, all the resentment, dismay, doubt and self-pity with which it is usually complicated.

C. S. Lewis, in a letter
to the grieving widower
Sheldon Vanauken

Despondent and dying of Hodgkin's disease, Matt lay in his hospital bed. Throughout his long illness, he had refused pastoral visits. He wanted no spiritual discussions. He had angrily insisted the Gideon Bible be removed from his room. He once had said, "Man created God. I created me."

He was in no physical pain, but seconds before his death, he sat bolt upright. Eyes blazing with fear, he screamed, "NO! NO! NO!" Then he fell back and died.

His wife wailed for over an hour, "Why? . . . It's not fair . . . I want him back . . . Why? . . ." No one could console her. A year later, grief still overwhelmed her. Five years later she had ovarian cancer.

That same week, I (DES) sat in another hospital room with a woman dying of breast cancer. She had suffered pain, but medication had kept it bearable. Here the atmosphere was very different.

I whispered in her ear. "It's time, Ruth. Is there anything more you want to say?"

She signaled for her husband to come over, and she mouthed the words, "I love you John. See you soon . . ."

"I love you, dear," he said, as he held her hand and kissed her cheek. She faded away while her pastor quietly read the twenty-third Psalm:

> The LORD is my shepherd; I shall not want. He maketh me to lie down in green pastures. . . . Yea, though I walk through the valley of the shadow of death, I will fear no evil: for thou art with me. . . . and I will dwell in the house of the LORD for ever. (KJV)

For a second I wondered if I sensed an angel, escorting her soul to heaven.

I will never forget the stark contrast between those two rooms. One family wept in hopeless heartache. The other wept with hopeful hearts. In one room, the flowers smelled of death. In the other, the prayers wafted like incense. One, a terrified man dropping into the unknown. The other, a restful soul passing through heaven's gate.

After sitting beside hundreds of deathbeds, we have seen this recurring pattern. People with a strong faith tend to die in peace. People without faith tend to die in terror and torment. This difference is not just our opinion. Studies have found that faith helps people cope with death. One study from the State University of New York found that among 115 elderly adults, "Religious subjects were . . . more prepared for death."[1] Another survey in the *Journal of Clinical Psychology* found that those with a devout faith "were significantly lower in death anxiety."[2]

When my (DES) wife visited Japan, a young Buddhist surgeon commented, "When I get old, I will become a Christian. . . . Only the Christians die with peace."

Thousands of years ago, Solomon made the same observation, "The righteous has hope in his death" (Prov. 14:32). Another wise man said, "Let me die the death of the righteous. Let my last be like his" (Num. 23:10).

Of Heartaches and Pain

Late one afternoon, I (SIM) walked up a quaint village sidewalk. The sun had painted a beautiful sunset mural, but I hardly noticed. I rang the doorbell and waited. Patti, a young housewife, cheerfully answered the door. "Hi, Doc. Come in. Have some orange juice. Jack should be home any . . ." Just then she noticed my somber frown. "Doc, what's wrong?"

"It's Jack," I said. "He had an accident on Route 19. He never knew what happened. There wasn't anything we could do."

Over the ensuing months, nonstop waves of grief poured over her, and she sank into a deep depression. If a lab had analyzed her blood, they would have found elevated stress hormones. These toxins so poisoned her body that her fingers soon became painful, swollen, and stiff. This arthritis progressed and finally crippled her.

Excessive grief can be dangerous. It may trigger ulcerative colitis, rheumatoid arthritis, heart attacks, and many other diseases. Within the first year after losing a spouse, widows and widowers are much more likely than other folks their age to die.

Today, while I (DES) was working on this chapter, a new patient made an urgent visit to my office. George was a confident, successful businessman; but today George was scared. "I'm not sure what's going on," he said. "I think maybe I had a heart attack."

The night before, while in bed watching TV, he gradually began to feel dizzy. His heart began fluttering. Sweat drenched his body. He developed chest pain and threw up. Then he went back to bed and fell asleep. Two hours later, he woke up, feeling wiped out. This was his third similar episode in the past three months.

When I questioned him, he did admit to being "under a lot of stress." He had recently moved cross-country, bought a house, and started a new business.

When I asked if he had any other big stresses, he mentioned that his twelve-year-old son had died in a car wreck two years earlier. "Since that day," he said, "nothing has been any fun." Every single minute of every single day, he thought of his dead son. He slept poorly and often awoke with nightmares. He found himself crying at the littlest thing.

George had suffered even more than the normal anguish of losing a child. His soul had plunged from sorrow to deep depression. He had tried counseling; it didn't help. He had divorced and remarried; life still felt empty. He had talked with a minister; it just "turned into an argument." Everywhere he had searched for relief, he had found only more pain. His emotions had become so twisted and tense that they had finally snapped in an anxiety attack. His chest pain came not from a heart attack but from a heartache.

Pain Relief or Healing

Losing a child always rips a gaping wound in the soul. Just as with physical wounds, wounds to the soul need healing. Too often, though, the modern psychiatrist gives only pills for pain relief.

Mere pain relief is a cop-out and borders on spiritual malpractice. If someone slices a hand with a bread knife, the doctor must wash and suture the wound. No sane doctor ignores the wound and just prescribes pain pills. Festering physical wounds don't heal and can even become cancerous. In the same way, wounds to the soul may fester and turn into the spiritual cancers of anger and depression.

A wound in the soul needs cleansing and healing. One must face it and deal with it. Spiritual healing works through pain to revitalize faith, hope, and peace.

Wherefore fear not,
    ye that have suffered;
For healing
    shall be your portion.
1 Enoch 96:3

Only spiritual healing can heal a wounded soul. Faith finds hope in Scripture. Faith finds comfort in the Holy Spirit. Faith finds meaning in prayer. God also often uses a community of faith—where people pray for each other, cry together, bring meals to the home, and simply say, "I heard about your loss. I'm sorry."

Again this benefit of faith is not just our opinion. The results of many studies agree. In one study, researchers followed 124 parents who had lost a baby to sudden infant death syndrome (SIDS). When they surveyed these people 18 months later, they found that people of faith had "greater well-being and less distress." These parents were more likely to have found meaning in their child's death and had received a greater social support in their loss.[3]

Without faith, parents often find the pain too great to face. With faith, they can eventually face the pain and experience hope. Then the wounded soul can begin to heal.

Death Defanged

When Lazarus fell ill, his family sent to Jesus for help. But Jesus seemed to dillydally until Lazarus had already died. Then he told his disciples that he was going merely to *"wake up"* Lazarus from a nap. No one in that culture ever spoke of "awakening" someone from the dead,[4] so the disciples were confused. Why would Jesus make a long journey into enemy territory just to wake up a sleeping man? Jesus saw that they were missing his point, so he spoke plainly: "Lazarus is dead" (John 11:14 NIV).

When Jesus finally arrived, Lazarus had been dead for four days. Jesus told the weeping Martha: "I am the resurrection and the life. He who believes in me will live, even though he dies. . . . Do you believe this?" (vv. 25, 26 NIV).

A million eloquent words would have convinced no one. But Jesus convinced many with three little words, "Lazarus, come out!" (v. 43 NIV). Out walked Lazarus, living proof that Jesus can *awaken* even the dead.

Children never worry whether parents can awaken them from sleep. In the same way, Christians can be sure that their

Lord will awaken them from *sleep.* This is the reason the early Christians renamed their graveyards "sleeping places" or *koimē-tērion,* the root for the English word *cemetery.*[5]

Once at another funeral everyone laughed at Jesus when he said of the corpse, "She's not dead; she's merely sleeping" (Luke 8:52). They thought he was a naive fool. But he wanted to teach them the true reality of the state we call *death,* so he merely took the girl's cold, limp hand and *awakened* her from the state he called *sleep.*

Paul also wrote to Christians whose loved ones had died: "We don't want you to stay ignorant about *those who are sleeping.* Then you won't grieve hopelessly like the rest of humanity" (1 Thess. 4:13).

Neither should we mourn today over our children, sleeping in their bedrooms. Of course, it is normal and healthy to shed tears over the separation caused by death. But Christians can take Jesus at his word. We need not grieve so inconsolably that we end up with attacks of arthritis and other diseases. From a biblical perspective, our sleeping loved ones have already *awakened* to the sound of Jesus' voice.

When Sheldon Vanauken was grief stricken over his wife's death, C. S. Lewis gently chided him in a letter, "Death—corruption—resurrection is the true rhythm: not the pathetic, horrible practice of mummification. Sad you must be at present. You can't develop a false sense of a duty to cling to sadness . . . when . . . sadness begins to vanish."[6]

Grief is natural and important—so important that psychologists speak of an "insufficient time of bereavement." Even Jesus became choked up and wept, when he saw the sorrow of Lazarus' family. If Jesus wept, surely we should weep. Indeed, bottled up sorrow can cause devastating disease. One writer put it this way, "the sorrow which has no vent in tears may make the other organs weep."[7]

A searching sorrow can smelt a purer, surer faith. Refining is never pleasant; but a refiner must pour dirty gold ore into a blazing fire. Out of the fire comes glistening gold. We admire the product but we shrink from the process.

A poet once spoke of the benefits of sorrow this way:

Sorrows are
  our best education.
A man can see farther through a tear
  than through a telescope.

Heaven's Hope

The question of the ages remains. If God is all-loving and all-powerful, why does God allow any sorrow? Wouldn't a loving God give us perfectly happy lives? The Bible's answer is, "Yes, but not yet."

Death and sorrow were not part of God's original plan; they resulted from our own human sin (1 Cor. 15:21; Rom. 6:23). Humanity, not God, is responsible for death. Even more, throughout this book we have seen how death and disease often directly result from specific sins.

Faith, however, looks beyond today's sorrows. Faith looks toward future promise: "God shall wipe away all tears from their eyes; and there shall be no more death, neither sorrow, nor crying, neither shall there be any more pain" (Rev. 21:4 KJV). Faith means that death is not a dead end but a gateway—a gateway to heaven.

I (SIM) wrote the original edition of *None of These Diseases* while I was going through a time of sorrow. Here is what I wrote.[8]

In December 1961 we received a letter that pierced our hearts, like an arrow shot from a midnight woods. Our daughter—a missionary in Zimbabwe, Africa—had been hospitalized for several weeks. A spinal tap had found an incurable yeast meningitis. Nine thousand miles from our home, our only child was dying.

Our grief might well have overwhelmed us if not for the comfort and solace of the Holy Spirit and the Bible. We wondered how people without Christ can bear such sorrow. More effective than any nerve pill, a biblical promise soothed our spirits: "For today's light trial is producing for us an immense weight of eternal glory; if we do not focus on the visible but on the unseen. For the visible things are temporary, but the unseen things are eternal" (2 Cor. 4:17–18).

This promise paints a clear picture of faith. Life is a balance. On one side lies a tiny ounce of lead—today's trouble. On the other side falls an "immense weight" of gold—"eternal glory."

My current load of sorrow seemed overwhelming. But God was turning "today's light trial" into "an immense weight of eternal glory." God—the divine Alchemist—was miraculously transforming our hearts of grieving lead into hopeful gold.

Heaven Can Weight

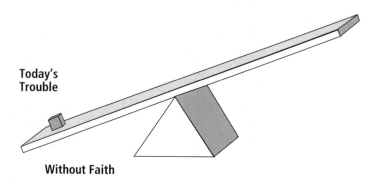

Today's Trouble

Without Faith

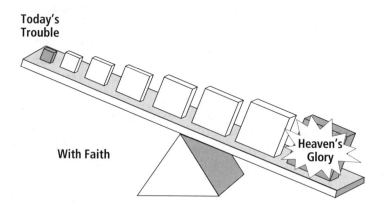

Today's Trouble

With Faith

Heaven's Glory

How could we have hope even in our sorrow? Watch the *"if"*—
"if we do not focus on the visible but on the unseen." The difference would depend on our disposition. Would we focus on today's troubles or tomorrow's destiny? Would we take an *earthbound* or a *heaven-bound* perspective?

Linda was *heaven-bound.* How could we mourn without accepting the solace of Scripture? Wouldn't we be selfish to mourn our own loss to the point of harming our own bodies? If our temporary loss would open heaven's gates for Linda, could true love mourn without finding comfort in her gain?

I love to think of my little children whom God has called to Himself as away at school—at the best school in the universe, under the best teachers, learning the best things, in the best possible way.
anonymous testimony of a bereaved parent

With time, sorrow always passes. It turns into either depression or hope. This depression is a long-term morbid preoccupation that persists for more than a year. Hope, on the other hand, is a long-term, appropriate confidence in the truth of God's promises. If we focused on today's sorrow, the sorrow would become depression. If, instead, we focused on future glory, God would transform sorrow into hope.

God blessed us with hope that could see farther through our tears than through any telescope: beyond today's troubles to tomorrow's glory—beyond this finite universe to an eternal heaven.

In the weeks that followed our daughter's letter, God's Word and Holy Spirit gave us a great peace. Sure, we were concerned but we also had hope. We had committed even her life into God's hands.

My daughter, her husband, and their two babies flew home. She came off the plane in a wheelchair. Her listless eyes sunken into her ashen face, she could hardly muster the effort to speak. I had seen many people with her look. Now, I knew the truth; Linda was dying.

> Doubt causes despair,
> > because it *focuses on the present*
> Faith gives hope,
> > because it *focuses on the future*.

Linda was admitted to a top medical center, where expert physicians searched for a diagnosis. White cells in her spinal fluid clearly signaled meningitis, but repeated spinal taps revealed no specific bacteria. Linda continued to languish with a low-grade fever, a severe headache, and persistent vomiting.

Her doctors tried several unproven treatments, but she continued her downward spiral. We began to accept the fact that she was dying. We still prayed for healing but we also found comfort in faith. If healing did not come, she would soon be with her Lord.

Then suddenly she started to get better. Her fever disappeared and her energy returned. One month later a spinal tap was normal in every respect. Was it in response to our prayers or an antibiotic? We believe that the answer is yes to both.

Will Linda's meningitis return when she stops the antibiotics? Is she cured, or has God granted only a temporary healing? We don't know. We don't know what the future holds, but we do know who holds the future.

Faith in God allows us to say with Paul: "Don't worry about anything, but in thankful prayers and petitions always give your concerns to God. And the peace of God, that is beyond human explanation will guard your hearts and minds in Christ Jesus" (Phil. 4:6–7).

Postscript

Linda did recover and she lived to walk once again through the valley of the shadow of premature death. In 1981 her doctors diagnosed a rare fatal cancer. She underwent radical surgery and one full year of grueling chemotherapy. Her hair fell out and she often felt nauseated. Her doctors gave her a 5 percent chance to survive five years. Again we looked to God and his promises. Once again God gave us his peace.

Still alive fifteen years later, Linda has far outlived her doctors' expectations. She has required four more major surgeries but she remains in good health. Has her medical treatment just postponed inevitable death from this cancer? Again we do not know what the future holds but we do know who holds the future.

At every family reunion, we thank the Lord, not for the sorrow itself and not just for Linda's physical healing. We thank God for the *result* of these experiences in the valley of the shadow of death. Through these experiences he has matured us and assured us of "an immense weight of eternal glory."

"Christians NEVER say good-bye!"
C. S. Lewis shouted this final farewell
to his dear friend Sheldon Vanauken
across a busy city street

Sorrows Like Sea Billows

H. G. Spafford, a successful Chicago businessman, experienced God's peace in the midst of great suffering. His wife and four of his five children were aboard an ocean liner, crossing the Atlantic, when their ship hit another vessel and began sinking. As panic struck the passengers, Mrs. Spafford gathered the children on deck. They prayed for deliverance but they also prepared their hearts to meet Jesus.

Within two hours, the ship along with the Spafford children had sunk under the dark Atlantic waters. Mrs. Spafford was saved by a passing boat. When she reached Cardiff, Wales, she telegraphed her husband two words, "Saved Alone."

Heartbroken, he set sail immediately to join his wife. One night the captain told Mr. Spafford, "I believe we are now passing over the spot where [the ship] went down. . . ." That night as Spafford looked out over the tossing ocean, these words flowed out of his aching heart:

When peace, like a river, attendeth my way,
When sorrows like sea billows roll;
Whatever my lot, Thou hast taught me to say,
It is well, it is well with my soul.

And Lord, haste the day when the faith shall be sight,
The clouds be rolled back as a scroll,
The trump shall resound and the Lord shall descend;
Even so—it is well with my soul.

It is well with my soul.
It is well, it is well with my soul.

This fleeting life may seem endearing. But through tears, we can gaze beyond this visible yet fleeting life and see farther than through a telescope. Through telescopes astronomers can see only millions of light years. Through tears we can see eternity.

TWENTY-SIX

Don't Shoot for the Moon

Vain the ambition of kings
Who seek by trophies
and dead things
To leave a living name
behind,
And weave but nets to
catch the wind.

John Webster,
The Devil's Law Case

"Daddy, I want to go to the moon." Those were the words of my (SIM) three-year-old daughter Linda as we sat on our open terrace in Africa. One could hardly blame her. The big tropical moon truly did look like you could reach up and touch the glowing globe of light. I carefully and patiently explained to her that the moon was much farther away than it appeared. No one had yet been able to go there.

Linda wanted to go so badly that she ignored all my explanations. She kept pleading excitedly. "Daddy, you don't even try. Go bring the dining table out here. Pile another table on it, and then all the chairs in the house, on top of each other." Exasperated with me, she stomped her feet and broke into tears.

When I recall her taut emotions, I can easily understand why shooting for the moon with all its frustrations often brings on disorders. There is a real relationship between *lunar* strivings and *lunacy*.

Arlene, a college senior, had been on the dean's list since her freshman year, a feat somewhat comparable to going to the moon. She loved seeing her name in that coveted column. But in her senior year she began to feel herself slipping. The thought of not achieving her goal made her anxious and panicky. She lost her ability to concentrate. She had already been accepted at a prestigious law school, so her grades meant little to her future career. Still she worried.

One day Arlene entered the infirmary because she couldn't read. She could pronounce words but could not understand what they meant. A week passed, no improvement. Each day she got more nervous, as those As got farther and farther from her reach.

She was sure there was something physically wrong with her. Even though I told her that she needed a changed viewpoint about striving for the moon, she continued to worry about her falling grades. She returned to her hometown, where she was thoroughly examined in a hospital. She was discharged with a large bill and a diagnosis of "somatic conversion disorder." In five-cent words, she was so emotionally upset that her mind couldn't read. Anxiety about her grades had produced a withdrawal symptom—an inability to read. She was unable to graduate with her class. She even lost her place in law school.

Banged, Battered, and Dented

Physical diseases often arise out of our desires to get to the top. The famous psychiatrist, Dr. Alfred Adler, taught that most psychological disorders arise from striving for power. The average Joe is caught in a daily struggle with others for power. No wonder his day is full of botched-up tasks, pent-up frustrations, messed-up feelings, and, often, banged-up fenders.

The next time you feel overly tired, stop and analyze the preceding hours. Ninety-nine times out of a hundred you will discover that someone recently let the air out of your ego. It is not our work that causes emotional and mental sluggishness and physical disease. Instead, these disorders often stem from trying to prove that our ideas are superior, our doctrines are truer, our church is better, our city is the choicest, our political party is the greatest, or our team is headed for the Super Bowl. Our, our, our—you name it, and we will argue with red faces that we are the people and that at our demise wisdom will surely vanish from the earth. It's a wonder we don't more often blow a cerebral fuse.

Once a young man came to my (SIM) office with a bloody eye. Nobody had punched him. A blood vessel had burst from forcing the high notes from his French horn. Remember his eye the next time you feel the need "to toot your own horn."

What a shame! Why do we race madly around life's oval like stock cars at Indy? We want to be first but we don't see the harm we're doing. In our race to be first, we bang, batter, and dent both ourselves and others.

Greatness—an Upside-Down View

Here are a few of the Bible's prescriptions, designed by God to save us from our blind ambitions. They would save millions of crushed and broken spirits if folks only had enough faith to apply them. How many of these prescriptions have you taken to heart?

- "Don't hold exaggerated ideas of yourself. Instead, have a sane estimate of who you are" (Rom. 12:3).
- "Love must be sincere. . . . Warmly love each other as family members. Honor each other above yourselves. . . . Do not be so highminded, but associate with lowly people. Do not be conceited" (Rom. 12:9, 10, 16).

- "Live in total harmony: one in love, one in soul, and one in thought. Never act in rivalry or for personal glory, but humbly think of each other before you think of yourselves" (Phil. 2:2–3).

At one time Jesus' disciples wanted to sit in places of authority and prominence. They argued about who would be the greatest in the kingdom. They even wanted to sit beside Jesus' throne in heaven. This power drive (what Dr. Adler called "ego ambition") controlled them. But they were embarrassed to ask Jesus about these things because they knew that Jesus had an upside-down view of greatness:

> [The scribes and pharisees] increase the size of their phylacteries and lengthen the tassels of their robes; they love seats of honor at dinner parties and front places in the synagogues. They love to be greeted with respect in public places and to have men call them "Rabbi!" Don't you ever be called "Rabbi"—you have only one teacher, and all of you are brothers. . . . And you must not let people call you "leaders"—you have only one leader, Christ! The only "superior" among you is the one who serves the others. For every man who promotes himself will be humbled, and every man who learns to be humble will find promotion.
>
> Matthew 23:5–12 Phillips

Jesus always challenges the world's philosophy. He warns against leadership aspirations.

Jesus' words would translate into college language as: Don't set your heart on being a four-pointer; don't sweat being homecoming queen; don't race to be class president, committee chairperson, or team captain. Graduate work may be needed, but don't do it to "lengthen the tassel" on the end of your name. The only "superior" among you is the one who serves the others.

Why does a four-point striver get sick, while another four-point student may suffer no injury? The striver seeks As for prestige and power. He is me-centered: me now, me first, me only . . .

If he refuses to adjust himself to humble situations, maybe his associates will decide to make the adjustments themselves. They will crudely chop his ego down to size. They may ruin his chemistry experiment. They won't help him study for a difficult test. They won't vote for him for class president. What irony! His striving to be first is the very thing that keeps him from it.

In contrast, practicing God's Word will spare you many bodily insults. The psalmist wrote, "Great peace have they who love your word, and nothing can upset them" (Ps. 119:165). Nothing? Not losing an election? Not getting a dreaded *A*-minus? Not being cut from the varsity team?

Everyone meets frustrating events every day, but the Christian need never get frustrated. I (SIM) saw college president Stephen W. Paine face several public embarrassments. Each time I was refreshed when he said, "It is perfectly all right. Perhaps the Lord sent it to keep me humble."

The Source of Security

The moon-shooter has only himself for security. The God-seeker finds security in God. The moon-shooter is like a self-employed store owner. When adversity hits, he has only his own resources to fall back on. A Walmart goes up down the street, and he must hold a going-out-of-business sale.[1]

But someone who is a vital part of a large corporation can rely on the resources of a Fortune 500 company. He has a sense of security. He knows that, no matter what happens tomorrow, the corporation is not likely to go bankrupt.

So is the man who is faithfully devoting his energies to the business of the King who owns the cattle on a thousand hills, the oil in a million wells, and the silver, gold, and jewels in a billion solar systems. In the benefits package of this King comes the security of absolutely guaranteed eternal life insurance. Not only is this man free from worries, insults, and antagonisms of self-seeking; but he can have a pleasing personality, denied to those who shoot for the moon.

Some time ago I read about a young woman who wanted to go to college. Her heart sank when she read one question on the application blank: "Are you a leader?" Being a conscientious girl she wrote "No" and sent in the form, but she was sure that she did not have a chance. To her surprise she received a letter from one of the college officials, which read something like this: "A study of our applications reveals that this year our college will have 1,452 freshmen leaders. Therefore, we are accepting you because we feel that they have need of at least one follower."

Always several hundred girls yearn to ride in the parade as the homecoming queen, but often only a half dozen show up to decorate the float. Construction crews never lack those who want to be job foreman but they have to search for men to drive nails and saw boards. Corporations have many would-be presidents, but few are happy to wash the office windows.

The whistling ditchdigger is more likely to dig the businessman's grave than to buy a coffin from him. Maybe, in our striving for the moon, we aren't too smart. I grant you, it must be a thrill to shoot for the moon in an upholstered space capsule. Yet, those original capsules bear an uncanny similarity to an asylum's padded cell.

Crucifying Self

Jesus said something that few people ever took seriously. He said, "The meek . . . will inherit the earth" (Matt. 5:5). We can believe that the meek will inherit heaven when they die, but Jesus also meant that the meek are going to inherit the earth here and now. Study the meek people you know and you will discover that they are actually coming into possession of everything that is worthwhile on this earth. Here is one of their prayers, seasoned with a bit of irony:

> Lord,
> Keep me from becoming verbose and
>   possessed with the idea
>   that I must express myself on every subject.

Release me from the craving
   to straighten out everyone else.
Teach me the glorious lesson that
   occasionally I may be wrong.
Make me helpful but
   not bossy.
With my vast store of wisdom and experience,
   it does seem a pity
   not to use it all.
But you know,
   Lord,
   that I want a few friends at the end.
Amen.

Jesus said, "The meek . . . will inherit the earth." Benito Mussolini and Adolf Hitler disagreed with this and tried to take the earth by force. They ended up with nothing.

How are we going to take care of this inner power urge, "the ego ambition"? Dr. Adler sought to appease this strong egotistical power urge and focus on helping others. He urged his patients to follow the Golden Rule: "Do to others what you would have them do to you" (Matt. 7:12 NIV).

The weakness of the Adler plan was that he was looking only at man's deviant power drive, which is only one symptom of our carnal nature. Freudian thought is similarly flawed in that it centers solely on another major carnal symptom—man's deviant sexual drive. The errors of both Adler and Freud lie in their merely treating *symptoms* of the carnal nature instead of treating the cause. When a person is dying of meningitis, it helps little to treat the symptoms of headache and fever with aspirin. The doctor must use antibiotics to attack the cause—the evil infection itself.

The Bible focuses therapy on the cause of the symptoms—the carnal nature: "People who belong to Christ Jesus have crucified the lower nature with its passions and desires . . ." (Gal. 5:24).

Instead of making frequent, expensive, and often futile trips to a psychiatrist's couch, Jesus invites us to share his cross and crucify our will. "While Christ was actually taking upon Himself the sins of humanity, God condemned that sinful nature" (Rom. 8:3). When you drive his nails into your selfish carnal nature, then God executes that old self of "ego ambition" and lustful attitudes. The road of death to self is the only way to new life in Christ.

"Jesus also suffered outside the city gate to make the people holy through his own blood. Let us, then, go to him outside the camp, bearing the disgrace he bore" (Heb. 13:12–13 NIV). Go outside the gate, beyond pompous human wisdom, and allow him to kill off the disease of self. Then you will be able to say with Paul, "I have been crucified with Christ: nevertheless I live; yet not I but Christ lives in me" (Gal. 2:20).

TWENTY-SEVEN

Are You Wearing a Parachute?

Christianity has not so much been tried and found wanting, as it has been found difficult and left untried.

G. K. Chesterton

What if you were a passenger on an airplane and the flight attendant handed you a backpack? What if she insisted you put it on, because it would make the trip more comfortable and fun? You would politely decline. If she forced you to wear it, you would soon be wiggling uncomfortably in your seat. You would feel cramped. Your back would ache. You would be irritated by the overbearing attendant.[1]

What if that same attendant handed you the same backpack, but this time she told you it was a parachute. She also told you that the plane was about to explode. Your only chance would be to jump. If you were not wearing the parachute, the law of gravity would condemn you to certain death. With that knowledge, you would strap on that pack with great appreciation. You wouldn't notice any discomfort. That lump in your back would feel like a snug hug. You would owe the flight attendant your life.

In the same way, if you try religion because someone tells you it will give you a "smoother flight," you will be disappointed. Your old friends may soon make fun of "Joe Religion." You may lose your job when you refuse to cheat a customer. Your minister may not be as entertaining as the one on TV. Serving others may eat into your time for golf or your favorite sitcom. This religion thing may seem more bothersome than a lumpy backpack on an airplane.

But the Christian life is not meant to saddle you with a bothersome backpack. In fact that lumpy backpack can feel as soft as a pillow. When is that backpack a comfy cushion? When you realize it is your only chance to be saved from death. When you realize that the law of gravity is against you.

Ten Great Cannons Pointed at You

Scripture states that we all have something much more serious than the law of gravity against us. We have the Law of God—the Ten Commandments. Which of the Ten Commandments have you violated? One? Two? Maybe three? Let's check.

   I. *"Love the Lord your God with all your heart."* Has anyone ever come between you and your love for God? Your lover? Your home? Your sports team? Your reputation?

   II. *"You shall not make any idol."* Do you ever imagine an all-loving God, who could never send anyone to hell? Have you thought that all roads lead to God? That may appear to be a wonderful concept, but is it true? Not according to God's Word. If you jump out of that airplane, and close your eyes believing that the clouds are cotton balls, will that erase the reality of gravity?

   III. *"Do not misuse God's name."* Have you ever said God's name in a casual way, using "God" as a sloppy substitute for "Wow!" or "Yeah!"? Worse yet, have you ever reduced

"God" to a curse word when you wanted to condemn someone to hell or you hit your thumb with a hammer?

IV. *"Observe the Sabbath day."* Have you always carefully honored God by setting aside special time to worship him?

V. *"Honor your father and mother."* Were you ever a teenager? Enough said.

VI. *"Do not murder."* Feel safe? Sorry. Scripture says that hating your neighbor is murder (1 John 3:15). Hate at the heart level is a wish (even for just a second) that the other person be obliterated from your world. It takes only a second to murder physically or emotionally.

VII. *"Do not commit adultery."* Have you ever lusted in your heart? If so, Jesus declares it a form of adultery (Matt. 5:28). Just as conspiracy (to burglary) breaks state law, so lust (for illicit sex) breaks God's moral law.

VIII. *"Do not steal."* Have you ever taken someone else's property, even when you knew no one would know? Ever fudged on your taxes? Ever gossiped and stolen someone's reputation?

IX. *"Do not testify falsely."* Have you ever shaded a story so that you looked even a little better and the other fellow looked a little worse?

X. *"Do not covet."* Have you ever been a little materialistic or greedy?

A little boy once asked his father, "What does it mean to covet?"

"It means," said the dad, "to really want something that is someone else's property."

"But Dad," said the boy, "everyone does that."

That's exactly the point. Those Ten Commandments—we have all broken every one. We may seem okay when graded on the curve by human standards. But by God's standards, we have failed in every conceivable way.

Scripture says that God is just. He must punish any and all violations of moral perfection. The punishment is hell—eternal separation from God.

"Wait one minute," you might say. "You're trying to lay a guilt trip on me."

All the Ten Commandments, like ten great cannons, are pointed at thee today, for you have broken all of God's statutes, and lived in daily neglect of all His commands. What will you do when the Law comes in terror, when the trumpet of the archangel shall tear you from your grave, when the eyes of God shall burn their way into your guilty soul, when the great books shall be opened, and all your sin and shame shall be punished?
Charles Haddon Spurgeon, 1834–1892

But maybe it's not so bad to feel guilty if you are guilty. Feeling guilt for wrongdoing is the only way for a criminal to begin to clean up his act. Feeling guilt for sin is the only way for a person to find cleansing for the soul.

Just as the law of gravity dictates the skydiver's destiny, the law of God points out your spiritual destiny. If you ignore the implications of the law of gravity, you are speeding at terminal velocity toward physical death. If you ignore the implications of God's moral law, you are rushing headlong into spiritual death. Scripture states, "The soul that sins, it shall die" (Ezek. 18:4). We are all lawbreakers. Death and destruction are our destiny.

On judgment day, no one will enter a plea of not guilty. We are all guilty. God cannot simply say, "You've been naughty, but I love you. Your rebellion isn't that big a deal. You did violate every command I ever gave, but I'll let it pass this time. It might be best if you don't let it happen again."

What a sham! What kind of God would treat his perfect moral law with such casual disdain? That would cheapen God's law and make it meaningless.

The One Exception

Everyone who has ever lived is guilty of violating God's law and deserves punishment. Everyone who has ever lived—except one. That one is Jesus. Jesus was not just a great man. He was a perfect man. He never violated a single line of God's law. He loved God perfectly. He always honored his parents. He never lied. He never sinned.

The men who testified to his perfection were eleven disciples who lived, slept, and ate with him. If he had moral defects, they would certainly have seen them. Jesus is the only man who ever lived who didn't deserve punishment. He didn't deserve to die yet he was brutally executed.

On judgment day God will simply declare every man and woman guilty. No one will argue the verdict. But there is a way out for those who have recognized their own guilt and have fled to God in repentance. For these, the punishment has been paid. Jesus died unjustly so that he could answer the justice of God and pay the penalty for your sins.

But I'm Pretty Good

"I'm not all that bad." This was the response of a young man with whom I (DES) had just shared this information.

"I know," I answered. "You're a great guy. But your relative goodness or badness is not the point. The question is this, 'Have you broken God's law?'"

"I guess so."

"What does that make you."

"A fudger?" he smiled.

"Nice try," I laughed. "A person who breaks the law is a . . ."

"Lawbreaker?"

"Very good. And lawbreakers deserve what?"

"Punishment?"

We cannot love God—cannot obey Him—and remain what we are. We must repent.

Charles W. Colson

"That's right. You're a lawbreaker. You deserve punishment. Compared to God's perfection, the Bible says your own goodness is like 'filthy rags.' Are you willing to trust your life to a parachute made of shredded filthy rags?"

"Maybe I need to rethink this a little."

The Answer

On judgment day no Johnny Cochran will concoct an emotional argument to sway a jury. No Norm Shapiro will shape a legal loophole to let you slip through. You will stand helpless and hopeless before a perfect, all-knowing God. Your conscience will be the prosecuting attorney. Your life will be the evidence. The judge will strike the gavel and declare: "Verdict: guilty. Sentence: death."

Your only hope is to have already staked your eternal destiny on what Jesus Christ did on the cross. Then Jesus, the Judge himself, will lovingly step away from the bench and take you in his arms and say: "Punishment: My child, I already paid it."

Death Leads to Life

What if you find that you agree with all of this, but in your heart it doesn't seem all that important? "I've never really felt sorry for my sin," you may say. "But I go to church. Anyways, what really matters is how I treat others." How you treat others does really matter. But if the story of Jesus' death seems irrelevant to your life, you may have never experienced the new life in Christ. If you have never shed a tear over your rebellion against God, it is unlikely that you have ever entered into the Christian life.

When you realize what Jesus has done for you, the cross will never seem trivial. Jesus didn't merely hand you a parachute. He didn't merely live a life that is a good example to follow. He suffered real torture, oozed real blood, and writhed in real pain—for you. If not for the sins of humanity, Jesus would not have needed to die. Your sins helped nail him to that cross. If one of those Roman soldiers hammering a nail into Jesus' hand were to turn and face you, you might be startled to see your own face on the body of that Roman soldier.

Many don't realize the seriousness of their own sin or the price that Christ paid on the cross. Christianity is just the religion they grew up in. They don't have anything against God. They are even willing to try to fit him into the corners of their life. They may even do God a few favors now and then: drop a few dollars in the offering, pray a short prayer (especially in a time of crisis), get a little emotional during a worship service, and maybe even mention that they go to church if someone asks.

[Here is] the very heart of repentance . . . that determination to forsake sin—to change one's attitude toward self, toward sin, and God; to change one's feelings: to change one's will. . . . There is not one verse of Scripture that indicates you can be a Christian and live any kind of a life you want to.

Billy Graham, *Peace with God*

But does this kind of Christian bear any likeness to a true Christ-follower? Jesus defined a Christian this way, "If anyone would come after me, he must first deny himself, take up his cross and follow me" (Matt. 16:24). When people came to Jesus, volunteering to be one of his faithful few, he rarely told them to "simply believe." Instead, he said, "Follow me." What he meant was that we are to repent. The word repent means to literally turn around and go the other way. Jesus called men and women to stop going their own way and to turn and make a radical commitment to walk as Jesus did.

You must not be like the man described in Scripture, who looked into the mirror of God's Word, saw how badly he needed a bath, and then didn't even take a Handywipe to his face (James 1:22–25). When you truly see the condition of your soul, you will recognize that a little rinse will never do. Your soul needs a complete bath.

When you realize the condition of your soul, when you realize the price that Jesus paid on the cross for you, when you realize that salvation involves not just a momentary decision but a life to be lived, then you are ready to repent.

Leave behind any halfhearted attitude—it's your whole heart or nothing. Give yourself fully to him. He will give himself fully to you.

Compared with the spiritual condition of your own soul, nothing else in this book has any importance or relevance. Forget physical wholeness, settle the spiritual issue first. Forget sexual wholeness, settle the spiritual issue first. Forget emotional wholeness, settle the spiritual issue first.

Once you have settled the spiritual issue, then you can move on and live the life God always intended for you. Then you can live in relationship with God. Then you can experience the blessings that he has in store for you.

TWENTY-EIGHT

The Soul Set Free

Each of us has heaven and hell in him.

Oscar Wilde,
The Picture of
Dorian Gray

One summer evening Joe Ransler went to the home of his brother, who was away working a night shift. He visited with his brother's wife, who, he later reported, "was dressed in shorts and a bra, like she always was." A few hours later, Joe had raped his sister-in-law. To hide his crime, he strangled both the woman and her little daughter. When Joe's brother came home the next morning, he found his wife and daughter dead.

After seven hours of questioning by the police, Joe confessed. "What makes a guy act like I do? I want to pray and everything and inwardly I feel that I want to be the best Christian in the world. But outwardly I'm a maniac and I can't control the outward part. I don't know why." He hadn't made much headway following the inward voice, for the police had previously arrested him a half dozen times. He did recognize, however, that in his soul a battle raged between two forces—one for good and one for evil. Robert Louis Stevenson dramatically illustrated our twofold nature in his novel about the man who was one moment the kindly Dr. Jekyll and the next moment the murderous Mr. Hyde.

The Conflict in Us

Dr. Karl Menninger recognized the existence of these two inner forces and referred to them as the "life instinct" and "death instinct." The life instinct seeks to preserve life; the death instinct seeks to destroy life. People standing near the brink of a deep canyon often sense the tug of both forces: one to jump, the other to step back. They usually heed the life instinct. Today's teens, however, live in a spiritual vacuum that has sapped them of the spiritual strength to win this struggle. This spiritual sickliness has resulted in thousands of teen suicides.

With a little self-inspection, each of us can sense the inner presence of the two opposing forces. Inside each of us, these forces battle a thousand times every day. When we are tempted to tell that little white lie to save face, an evil force whispers, "Everybody does it. No one will know the difference." When we are tempted to pass on that juicy tidbit of slanderous gossip, that evil force can seem irresistible. We haven't had to hang by the neck for murder, but many times we should have hung our faces for shame.

The famous psychiatrists Freud, Adler, and Jung largely agreed that most mental illness arises from psychological conflict between good and evil forces. Freud emphasized the sexual perversions of the bad force. Adler stressed its ruthless drive for power. Jung likened the evil force to a wild, ravenous wolf. Jung even noted that neuroses arise from the battle between these two forces. "The conflict may be between the sensual and the spiritual man. . . . [Thus] healing may be called a religious problem."[1]

Of course this battle results not only in psychological diseases but in physical diseases as well, caused by envy, jealousy, self-centeredness, resentment, fear, and hatred. These are the same emotions that the Bible lists as arising from the evil force within us.

The Battle Is Spiritual

Psychologists and psychiatrists have recognized this conflict but they tend to attribute problems arising from this conflict to "poor ego strength" or chemical imbalance. They mostly ignore the fact that it is a spiritual battle for your soul. Most of psychiatry doesn't realize that today's epidemics of neurosis, anxiety, and depression are a direct result of the spiritual malaise of the modern world.

Dr. Carl Jung, however, recognized the spiritual aspect of disease and healing:

> During the past thirty years, people from all the civilized countries of the earth have consulted me. I have treated many hundreds of patients. . . . Among all my patients in the second half of life—that is to say, over thirty-five—there has not been one whose problem in the last resort was not that of finding a religious outlook on life. . . .
>
> It seems to me, that, side by side with the decline of religious life, the neuroses grow noticeably more frequent. . . .
>
> The patient is looking for something that will take possession of him and give meaning and form to the confusion of his neurotic mind. Is the doctor equal to the task? To begin with, he will probably hand over his patient to the clergyman or the philosopher, or abandon him to that perplexity which is the special note of our day. . . . Human thought cannot conceive any system or final truth that could give the patient what he needs in order to live: that is faith, hope, love and insight. . . .
>
> There are however persons who, while well aware of the psychic nature of their complaint, nevertheless refuse to turn to the clergyman. . . . It is from the clergyman, not from the doctor, that the sufferers should expect such help.[2]

Since my evil nature is a spiritual problem, the battle against it is not medical or psychological. It is spiritual. No wonder mere counseling and medications can't free me from it.

The Picture of You and Me

Oscar Wilde described this evil force in his novel, *The Picture of Dorian Gray*. As a young Adonis, Dorian sits for a painted portrait. Later he stares at his incredibly handsome likeness and he is stung with the realization that his portrait will be forever young and handsome, but in a few short years his body will age and shrivel. Dorian quips that he would trade his soul to stay eternally young but he never expects his flippant wish to be granted.

One day, however, he discovers that his adoring fiancée is not the perfect goddess that he had naively fantasized, so he angrily dumps her. Brokenhearted, she commits suicide. The next day he glances at his portrait and suspects he sees a leering ugliness forming in the picture. As the years pass he hurts more and more people, and the picture disfigures more and more grotesquely. It is the reflection of his very soul.

Disgusted by his horrid inner self, he hides the picture in his attic. He lives in constant fear that someone, anyone, will break into the attic and catch a glimpse of his wretched soul. Still, the picture fascinates him; and he frequently steals away into the locked attic, uncovers his shameful reflection, and stares.

We [should] . . . lay a clear constant emphasis upon the cost of *non*-discipleship . . . a life of crushing burdens, failures, and disappointments, a life caught in the toils of endless problems that are never resolved . . . that unending soap opera, that sometimes horror show known as normal human life.

Dallas Willard, *The Spirit of the Disciplines*

The picture finally destroys Dorian. His fear and revulsion lead him to murder the portrait artist and slash the picture with a knife. But when he shreds the picture, he annihilates his soul. Instantly he ages and dies.

The Bible says that your evil nature will spiritually destroy you in the same way. Your only hope is to allow Christ to destroy it.

Religious Life

Many today don't want to deal with their own evil nature; they would rather just try to feel good and ignore their spiritual health. They may try the latest fad in spirituality.

They may also apply this same wishful thinking to their physical health. They don't want to change their exercise habits; they want a "miracle" anti-aging diet. They don't want to change their prayer habits; they want the "miracle" stress vitamin. They don't want to change their eating habits; they want the "miracle" weight-loss herb.

They want the blessings of "none of these diseases" without following the teachings of Jesus. They want freedom from misery but they don't want to crucify anger. They want healing from neurosis but they don't want to give up their self-centeredness. They want joy unspeakable but they still want to gossip. In short, they want the impossible. They want the blessings of the victorious Christian life without living a Christian life.

This is why churches are full of people who find religion frustrating and unfulfilling. They make a halfhearted commitment to God but they expect a wholehearted commitment from God to meet their every need. Their faith might be called a "what-can-I-get-away-with" faith.

People with this halfhearted attitude miss out on so much. They miss the blessings of the new life. They miss real joy. They miss real peace. They miss all the blessings described throughout this book. Jesus himself had no patience for what-can-I-get-away-with followers. He said that he would spit out an uncommitted Christian like a mouthful of lukewarm coffee (Rev. 3:16).

Power to Change

Your selfish evil nature is no different than Dorian Gray's. The Bible says, "Lurking within you is . . . sexual immorality, impurity, lust, shameful passions, and greed . . . anger, rage, hate, gossip, and filthy talk . . . lying" (Col. 3:5, 8, 9).

Your selfish self is as much a part of you as a shell is of a turtle. Escape seems impossible. Nineteen centuries before the birth of psychiatry, Paul described his natural state—in the clutches of an evil force:

> My own behavior baffles me. For I find myself not doing what I really want to do but doing what I really loathe. Yet surely if I do things that I really don't want to do, I am admitting that I really agree with the Law. But it cannot be said that "I" am doing them at all—it must be sin that has made its home in my nature. (And indeed, I know from experience that the carnal side of my being can scarcely be called the home of good!) I often find that I have the will to do good, but not the power. That is, I don't accomplish the good I set out to do, and the evil I don't really want to do I find I am always doing. . . . It is an agonizing situation, and who on earth can set me free from the clutches of my own sinful nature?
>
> Romans 7:15–20, 24 Phillips

Like a man in a straitjacket, Paul had found that he could not squirm free from his selfish evil nature.

But then Paul met Jesus and he experienced life-changing power. God filled Paul with a spiritual force much stronger than his evil nature. Suddenly God gave him the power to change from the inside out:

> Thank God that there is a way out through Jesus Christ our Lord. . . . God sent his own Son in human likeness, so that he could put to death the evil force in humanity. . . . So if Christ lives in you, the evil nature is dead because *Jesus has conquered* sin; and the Spirit in you is alive because of *Jesus'* righteousness.
>
> Romans 7:25; 8:3, 10

When Jesus died on the cross, "Our old self was crucified with him, so that our evil nature might be destroyed. We are no longer slaves to sin, because when we died with Christ we were set free from sin" (Rom. 6:6–7). The Spirit of Christ living in us fills us with spiritual power to win this spiritual battle. "If you kill off your instinctive evil nature by obeying the Spirit, you are truly alive" (Rom. 8:13).

Those old habits, those old practices, those old attitudes—they all must go. You may feel a twinge of remorse as the casket closes on your old way of life, for it has given you many of life's so-called pleasures. But remember, you are not saying good-bye to worthwhile pleasures but to pleasures that are a death force. As with Dorian Gray, later they will bring you only pain. Jesus has something much better in mind for you:

> I promise you . . . nobody leaves home or brothers or sisters or mother or father or children or property for my sake and the Gospel's without getting back a hundred times over, now in this present life . . . and in the next world eternal life.
>
> Mark 10:30–31 Phillips

Jesus promises, even here "in this present life," "a hundred times" more of the truly worthwhile—including healthy habits and healthy attitudes.

> Jesus not only saved me from my guilt and my sin, he saved me from me.
>
> Dennis Kinlaw

This crucifixion of your old way of life is not a once-and-for-all event, but a daily process—a process of self-inspection, repentance, receiving forgiveness, and renunciation of sin. This crucifixion is a daily funeral for your death instinct and a daily realization of your new birth in Christ.

Prior to your new birth, you were powerless to escape from the domination of your evil nature. Prior to his new birth, even the great apostle Paul had thrown up his hands in frustration: "What a wretched man I am! Who can set me free from the clutches of my deadly evil nature?" (Rom. 7:24). This is the greatest human question of all time. Both Saint Paul and the sex murderer Ransler faced it.

There is no lack of answers. Every psychiatric school has a different one—pretty good evidence that none is truly effective. Worse yet, these various schools concern themselves with merely treating symptoms. They ignore the spiritual nature of the battle for your soul, so they never get to the root of the problem.

Only the Bible deals with the spiritual root of your problem.

> If we have been united with him like this in his death, we will certainly also be united with him in his resurrection. For we know that our old self was crucified with him so that the body of sin might be done away with, that we should no longer be slaves to sin.
>
> Romans 6:5–6 NIV

For Jesus, the path to resurrection had to go right through the cross. For you, it is the same. Your path to new life runs right through the cross. Every day you must escort your selfish, evil nature to the cross and there watch it die. Then you can experience the resurrection life in Christ.

- Death to self is the only way to inner peace.
- Death to self is the only way to true spirituality.
- Death to self is the only way to deep joy.
- Death to self is the only way to claim God's promise, "none of these diseases. . . ."

Appendix

Infant Circumcision: A Guide for Parents

As with all medical procedures, give consent for circumcision only after you have a frank discussion of the risks and benefits with your doctor. Loving parents may decide for or against infant circumcision. Modern doctors can treat most problems associated with either circumcision or uncircumcision. Make the decision that seems best for you and your boy.

When *Not* to Circumcise

A. If your doctor finds an abnormality that may need to be repaired using the foreskin, do not have your son circumcised. Ask your doctor if you have any questions.
B. Never allow circumcision on a sick or premature baby.
C. If you have difficulty accepting responsibility for risk, maybe you should decide not to circumcise. We believe the benefits outweigh the risks, but some doctors disagree. Circumcision complications (including infection, bleeding, and deformity) occur rarely (about 2 per 1,000). They

are usually, but not always, easily treated. Three deaths due to circumcision have been reported since 1954. To put this in perspective, by our calculations, a baby is more likely to die on the car ride home from the hospital than from a circumcision complication. Discuss the risks with your doctor.

D. Consider avoiding circumcision if you fear that it may result in long-standing psychological harm to you or to the boy.

E. If both parents cannot agree, we recommend not circumcising the boy.

The Risks and the Benefits

	Against Circumcision	*For Circumcision*
Death	Three reported deaths due to circumcision in almost 30 years.	Annually, without circumcision, urinary tract infection (UTI) complications might result in up to 60 infant deaths; penile cancer in about 750 adult deaths.
Pain	All boys experience pain, if only from the local anesthetic injection.	Greater and longer-lasting pain for up to 10 percent of men* who will need circumcision later in life.
Surgical Complications	About 2 per 1,000 circumcisions have complications —mostly simple bleeding and minor infections. Severe complications are very rare.	If no boys were circumcised, we estimate up to 60 infants might suffer renal failure and 90 might suffer meningitis annually from UTI complications.
Penile Problems	More common in uncircumcised boys.	Rare in circumcised boys. However, disfigured genitals can result from

	Against Circumcision	For Circumcision
		complications or errors in technique.
Sexually Transmitted Disease	Two studies have suggested a lower rate for an STD in uncircumcised men.	Almost 50 studies have shown that circumcision protects against many different STDs: and a 2- to 10-fold protection against HIV.
Cost	Annual cost for circumcising all infant boys is $250 million.*	If no infant circumcision, annual cost for later circumcision of up to 10 percent of all males is $400 to 800 million.*
Chronic Diseases	Lack of circumcision is not known to protect against any chronic disease.	Annually, without circumcision, UTI complications might result in 2,000 cases of kidney scarring and 500 cases of hypertension or renal failure.*

Note: These are rough estimates for the United States based on currently available data.

Should We Circumcise to Be Good Christians?

For Christians, circumcision has no religious significance. The New Testament clearly states that physical circumcision is not required (Gal. 5:1–6; 1 Cor. 7:17–20). Circumcision is a religious rite for members of the Jewish and Islamic faiths.

If You Decide to Circumcise:

A. Find a doctor who has performed hundreds of circumcisions. If you are in a hospital using physicians in training, you may request the attending physician to be physically present during the procedure.

B. To reduce pain, you may request an anesthetic nerve block. Some doctors, however, prefer not to use this technique until it is proven safe in a large study.

C. After the procedure, hold and console your baby. Most parents marvel at how quickly their baby recovers.

If You Decide against Circumcision:

A. Many informed, caring parents decide against circumcision. It may be best for you.

B. Talk with your baby's doctor to learn how gently to retract and wash the foreskin. Later, teach the boy how to do it himself.

C. Your boy may need circumcision later if he develops trouble with inflammation or an unretractable foreskin.

Further Research

For further reading, we suggest editorials by Dr. Thomas Wiswell (pro-circumcision) and Dr. Thomas Metcalf (anti-circumcision), "Do You Favor Routine Neonatal Circumcision?" *Postgraduate Medicine* 84, no. 5 (October 1988): 98–108. Your hospital librarian or public library should be able to get a copy.

Notes

Chapter 1   *Eel Eyes and Goose Guts*

1. S. E. Massengill, *A Sketch of Medicine and Pharmacy* (Bristol, Tenn.: S. E. Massengill, 1943), 16.

2. As quoted by Guido Manjo, *The Healing Hand: Man and Wound in the Ancient World* (Cambridge, Mass.: Harvard University Press, 1975), 102.

3. Ibid.

Chapter 2   *Back to the Breakthrough*

1. George Rosen, *A History of Medicine* (New York: MD Publications, 1958), 62–63.

2. Ibid., 63–65.

3. *The Edwin Smith Surgical Papyrus,* trans. James H. Breasted (Chicago: University of Chicago Press, 1930), 473–75.

4. Ibid., 15.

5. Arturo Castiglione, *A History of Medicine* (New York: Alfred A. Knopf, 1941), 71.

6. Th. M. Vogelsang, "Leprosy in Norway," *Medical History* 9 (1965): 31.

7. C. C. Shepard, "The Nasal Excretion of *Mycobacterium leprae* in Leprosy," *International Journal of Leprosy* 30 (1962): 10.

8. K. V. Desikan, "Viability of *Mycobacterium leprae* Outside the Human Body," *Leprosy Review* 48 (1977): 231.

9. Rosen, *A History of Medicine,* 63–65.

Chapter 3   *A Labor of Love*

1. The exact medical term is *puerperal fever* or *puerperal sepsis.*

2. One exception was smallpox, which was considered to be a contagious disease.

3. Literally, "unclean."

4. I. E. S. Edwards, "Mummy," *The Academic American Encyclopedia* (electronic version), (Danbury, Conn.: Grolier, 1992).

5. As quoted in Ignaz Semmelweis, *Die Ætiologie,* trans. F. P. Murphy, *Medical Classics* 5 (1941): 560.

6. Semmelweis, *Die Ætiologie.*

7. A. C. Steere and G. F. Mallison, *Annals of Internal Medicine* 83 (1975): 685.

8. Actually it contains the isomer of thymol, carvacrol. The hyssop of biblical times is thought to be a type of marjoram.

9. *An Epitome of the History of Medicine*, 2nd ed. (Philadelphia: F. A. Davis, 1901), 326.

10. John P. Burke et al. *"Proteus Mirabilis* Infections in a Hospital Nursery Traced to a Human Carrier," *New England Journal of Medicine* 284 (1971): 115.

Chapter 4   *To Sewer or Not to Sewer*

1. Sanitary Report, p. 31, as cited by R. A. Lewis, *Edwin Chadwick and the Public Health Movement: 1832–1854* (London: Longmans, Green & Co., 1952), 47. We are deeply indebted to Lewis's work, without which most of the information in this chapter would be unavailable.

2. *Times,* 5 July 1849, as cited by Lewis, *Chadwick,* 221.

3. *Times,* 24 October 1848, as quoted by Lewis, *Chadwick,* 190.

4. *Second Report of the Metropolitan Sanitary Commission,* p. 22; P.P., 1847–48, vol. xxxii, p. 253.

5. Quoted by Chadwick and cited by Lewis, *Chadwick,* 244.

6. Quoted by Lewis, *Chadwick,* 244.

7. Literally, "Board of Guardians."

8. Summarized by Lewis, *Chadwick,* 192.

9. Quoted by J. H. Harley Williams, *A Century of Public Health in Britain: 1832–1929* (London: A & C Black, 1932), 268.

10. Chadwick, letter to Andrew Boardman, quoted by Lewis, *Chadwick,* 333.

11. *Third Report of the Metropolitan Sanitary Commission,* p. 14; P.P., 1847–48, vol. xxxii, p. 339, as quoted by Lewis, *Chadwick,* 219.

12. "Centralisation or Representation?" (1848), ix, as cited by Lewis, *Chadwick,* 167.

13. E. Hodder, *Observer* ii, p. 296, as quoted by Lewis, *Chadwick,* 215.

14. Lewis, *Chadwick,* 3.

15. Thomas Winset with Melanie Findig, *Backpacking Basics* (Berkeley, Calif.: Wilderness Press, 1988), 87–88.

16. Castiglione, *A History of Medicine,* 70.

17. Charles C. J. Carpenter, "Cholera" in *Harrison's Principles of Internal Medicine,* 11th ed. (New York: McGraw Hill, 1987), 619.

Chapter 5   *A Cemetery Plot*

1. *Report of Interment in Towns,* 31, as cited by Lewis, *Chadwick,* 69.

2. *Report of Interment in Towns,* 38, as summarized by Lewis, *Chadwick,* 69.

3. *Report of Interment in Towns,* 135, as quoted by Lewis, *Chadwick,* 73.

4. *Report of Interment in Towns,* 31, as cited by Lewis, *Chadwick,* 71.

5. Quoted by Chadwick in a letter cited by Lewis, *Chadwick,* 244.

6. Hansard, vol. cxxxv, 980–94, as quoted by Lewis, *Chadwick*, 365.

7. Quoted in Williams, *A Century of Public Health in Britain*, 268.

8. *Daily News*, 7 July 1890, as quoted by Lewis, *Chadwick*, 374.

9. This direction was given in the context of capital punishment. In practice, rapid burial was the norm and the biblical injunction applies this even to the executed criminal. This is borne out by later Jewish tradition where burial was always on the same day in Jerusalem and within three days elsewhere.

10. John 11:17 notes that Lazarus was "already entombed for four days," and John 11:39 notes that he would smell since it was "four days [since his death]." *Note:* John 11:39 would not be referring to time in the tomb, for it is time since death that will determine the level of decomposition and stench of the corpse. Thus Lazarus also appears to have been buried on the day of his death. Also, the record of Jesus' same-day burial reaffirms this interpretation.

Chapter 6   *Beelzebub in a Bottle*

1. Secretary of Health and Human Services, *Fourth Special Report of the U.S. Congress on Alcohol and Health* (Washington, D.C.: Government Printing Office, 1981).

2. U.S. Department of Health and Human Services, *First Statistical Compendium on Alcohol and Health* (Washington, D.C.: Government Printing Office, 1981).

3. A. Medhus, "Mortality among Female Alcoholics," *Scandinavian Journal of Social Medicine* 3 (1975): 111.

4. *Macbeth*, II, iii., 34.

5. Institute of Medicine, *Alcoholism and Related Problems: Opportunities for Research* (Washington, D.C.: National Academy of Sciences, 1980).

6. Alcoholics Anonymous, *Big Book of AA*, 3d ed. (New York: Alcoholics Anonymous World Services, Inc., 1976), 7. Text of first edition available on many Internet sites; search: + "Alcoholics Anonymous" + "Big Book."

7. Ibid., 9.

8. Ibid., 10.

9. Ibid., 11.

10. This was seen as only "a beginning." At first, "surrender to whatever you know about [God]" (Samuel Shoemaker, *The Conversion of the Church* [New York: Fleming Revell, 1932], 128), and move forward from there was the original idea behind "God, as I understand him." Later many corrupted this to mean "God, as I want him to be." Thus one's "Higher Power" is sometimes absurdly stated as a tree, Santa Claus, or a stuffed animal. This profane frivolity condemns the alcoholic to failure.

11. These five *C*s were part of the Oxford Group formula for seeing one's need and using God's power to save. Rev. Shoemaker clearly espoused these

elements as can be seen in his book, *Realizing Religion* (New York: Association Press, 1923), appendix 1.

12. Samuel Shoemaker, *If I Be Lifted Up* (New York: Fleming Revell, 1931), 83.

13. Sam saw A.A. not as a spiritual end in itself but rather a "precursor to the Church." Speech to A.A.'s Third International Convention, Long Beach, Calif., 3 July 1960, as cited in Dick B., *New Light on Alcoholism: The A.A. Legacy from Sam Shoemaker* (Kihei, Maui, Hawaii: Paradise Research Publications, 1998), 139. Bill Wilson himself often called A.A. a "spiritual kindergarten" (Dick B., *New Light*, 8).

14. Two citations of this phrase "born again" have been located in Bill's original manuscripts but they were removed from published accounts, as noted by Dick B., *New Light*, 37, footnote 10.

15. Alcoholics Anonymous, *Big Book*, 13.

16. Shoemaker, *Realizing Religion*, 21.

17. Samuel Shoemaker, *National Awakening* (New York: Harper & Brothers, 1936), 57–58.

18. See http://www.dickb.com/archives/aa_roots.html for a review of the book *Dr. Bob and the Good Oldtimers* (New York: Alcoholics Anonymous World Services, 1980).

19. Bill Wilson, *The Language of the Heart: Bill W.'s Grapevine Writings* (New York: The A.A. Grapevine, Inc.), 198.

20. *Alcoholics Anonymous Comes of Age* (New York: Alcoholics Anonymous World Services, Inc., 1957), 39–40.

21. We are indebted for much of the information in this chapter to Dick B. who has authored many books detailing his encyclopedic research into the Christian origins of A.A. These books may be ordered at www.dickb.com. The somewhat confused doctrines of A.A. have been amply pointed out by Tim Stafford, "The Hidden Gospel of the 12 Steps," *Christianity Today* (22 July 1991).

22. Alcoholics Anonymous, *Big Book*, 53, 181, 59.

23. Samuel Shoemaker, speech to A.A.'s Third International Convention, as cited by Dick B., *New Light*, 139.

24. Shoemaker, *Realizing Religion*, 9.

Chapter 7 *Cancer by the Carton*

1. Alton Ochsner, *Smoking and Cancer* (New York: Julian Messner, 1954), 12.

2. G. Hammond and L. Garfinkel, "General Air Pollution and Cancer in the United States," *Preventive Medicine* 9 (1980): 206.

3. N. L. Benowitz et al., "Smokers of Low-Yield Cigarettes Do Not Consume Less Nicotine," *New England Journal of Medicine* 309 (1983): 139; J. H. Jaffe et al., "Carbon Monoxide and Thiocyanate Levels in Low Tar/Nicotine Smokers," *Addictive Behaviors* 6 (1981): 337.

4. D. W. Kaufman et al., "Nicotine and Carbon Monoxide Content of Cigarette Smoke and the Risk of Myocardial Infarction in Young Men," *New England Journal of Medicine* 308 (1983): 409.

5. Complaint filed by *State of Kansas vs. R. J. Reynolds et al.*, District Court of Shawnee County, Kansas, case no. 96-CV, #133–146.

6. H. W. Daniell, "Smokers' Wrinkles: A Study in the Epidemiology of 'Crow's Feet,'" *Annals of Internal Medicine* 75 (1971): 873.

7. L. D. Johnson, J. G. Bachman, and P. M. O'Malley, *National Survey Results on Drug Use from the Monitoring the Future Study: 1975–1997* (Ann Arbor, Mich.: Institute for Social Research, 1998). Reported prevalence, 1991=17.9 percent and 1997=23.6 percent.

8. *State of Kansas vs. R. J. Reynolds et al;* Andrew Tisch, #43.

9. M. A. Russel, P. V. Cole, and E. Brown, "Absorption by Non-Smokers of Carbon Monoxide from Room Air Polluted by Tobacco Smoke," *Lancet* 1 (1973): 576.

10. www.cdc.gov/od/oc/media/fact/smoketsc.htm

11. This and much more data on secondhand smoke is available at web site: www.cdc.gov/tobacco

12. N. R. Butler and H. Goldstein, "Smoking in Pregnancy and Subsequent Child Development," *British Medical Journal* 4 (1973): 573.

13. J. Goujard, C. Rumeau, and D. Schwartz, "Smoking During Pregnancy: Stillbirth and *Abruptio Placentae*," *Biomedicine* 23 (1975): 20–22.

14. Surgeon General, *Health Consequences of Smoking for Women* (Washington, D.C.: Government Printing Office, 1980), 192.

15. K. C. Schoendorf and J. L. Kiely, "Relationship of Sudden Infant Death Syndrome to Maternal Smoking during and after Pregnancy," *Pediatrics* 90 (1992): 905–8.

16. www.cdc.gov/tobacco/who/usa.htm

17. *Journal of the American Medical Association* (18 November 1998).

18. Complaint filed by *State of Kansas vs. R. J. Reynolds et al.*, #186.

19. J. Forbes Moncrief, *Our Boys and Why They Should Not Smoke* (Manchester: British Anti-Tobacco and Anti-Narcotic League, circa. 1900), as cited at www.forces.com/pages/forest01.htm

20. B. Mausner and E. S. Platt, *Smoking: A Behavioral Analysis* (New York: Pergamon Press, 1971).

21. Complaint filed by *State of Kansas vs. R. J. Reynolds et al.*, #203.

22. James Johnston, before Congressional hearings in 1994. Complaint filed by *State of Kansas vs. R. J. Reynolds et al.*, # 43.

23. Thomas Sandefur, CEO for Brown and Williamson, before the House Energy and Commerce Subcommittee on Health and the Environment, then chaired by Henry Waxman.

24. Addison Yeaman, before Congressional hearings in 1994, as quoted in Complaint filed by *State of Kansas vs. R. J. Reynolds et al.*, #42.

25. J. L. Hamilton, *Review of Economics and Statistics* 54 (1972): 401.

26. The Pooling Project Research Group, *Journal of Chronic Diseases* 31 (1978): 201.

27. H. M. Annis, "Patterns of Intra-Familial Drug Use," *British Journal of Addiction* 69 (1974): 361.

28. Complaint filed by *State of Kansas vs. R. J. Reynolds et al.*, #126.

29. Ibid., #128.

30. E. Jones, *Sigmund Freud: Life and Work*, 3 vols. (London: Hogarth Press, 1953), 339.

31. R. A. Krumholz, R. B. Chevalier, and J. C. Ross, "Change in Cardiopulmonary Functions Related to Abstinence from Smoking," *Annals of Internal Medicine* 62 (1965): 197–207.

32. www.cdc.gov/od/oc/media/fact/smok1995.htm

33. Surgeon General, *Smoking and Health* (Washington, D.C.: Government Printing Office, 1979), chap. 22, p. 10.

34. www.cdc.gov/tobacco/who/usa.htm

35. Quoted in Count Egon Corti, *A History of Smoking*, trans. Paul England (London: George G. Harrap, 1931), 103.

36. Ibid., 119.

37. Quoted in Sean Gabb, *Smoking and Its Enemies: A Short History of 500 Years of the Use and Prohibition of Tobacco* (London: Freedom Organisation for the Right to Enjoy Smoking Tobacco, 1900).

38. Quoted in Gerald S. Lestz, *Tobacco: Pro and Con* (Lancaster, Pa.: Aurand Press, 1989), 11.

39. Moncrief, *Our Boys and Why They Should Not Smoke*.

40. Islam and modern Judaism would be partial exceptions. These exceptions, however, prove the rule. The Old Testament is Scripture for both Christians and Jews; and Mohammed borrowed much theology from Judaism and Christianity. Thus these exceptions actually support the miraculous uniqueness of the Bible. Only those religions with some sort of biblical roots have this concept that the body matters to God.

Chapter 8   *Torture or Nurture?*

1. Rosemary Romberg, *Peaceful Beginnings* (Anchorage: Peaceful Beginnings, 1982), 6.

2. Rosemary Romberg, *The "Heart" of the Matter* (S. Hadley, Mass.: Bergin & Garvey, 1988).

3. Terry Schultz, "A Nurse's View on Circumcision," *Mothering* 12 (1979): 83.

4. John Erickson, "Some Statements about Circumcision by Circumcised Men" (Anchorage: Peaceful Beginnings, 1988).

5. Rosemary Romberg, *Circumcision: The Painful Dilemma* (S. Hadley, Mass.: Bergin & Garvey, 1985).

6. Quoted by Dave Barry, "Circumcisions beyond Our Control," *Washington Post Magazine* (8 December 1991), 48.

7. *Hippocrates* (February 1993): 53.

8. Dave Barry's "Circumcisions beyond Our Control" gave me the idea to ask these questions, and my results were almost identical to his.

9. American Academy of Pediatrics, *Committee on Fetus and Newborn: Standards and Recommendations for Hospital Care of Newborn Infants,* 5th ed. (Evanston, Ill.: American Academy of Pediatrics, 1971).

10. W. K. C. Morgan, "The Rape of the Phallus," *Journal of the American Medical Association* 193 (1965): 223.

11. W. K. C. Morgan, "Penile Plunder," *Medical Journal of Australia* 7 (1967): 1102.

12. T. E. Wiswell, "Prepuce Presence Portends Prevalence of Potentially Perilous Perurethral Pathogens," *The Journal of Urology* 148 (1992): 739; grammar corrected.

13. T. E. Wiswell and J. D. Roscelli, "Corroborative Evidence for the Decreased Incidence of Urinary Tract Infections in Circumcised Male Infants," *Pediatrics* 78 (1986): 96.

14. Nicholas Cunningham, "Circumcision and Urinary Tract Infections," *Pediatrics* 77(1986): 267.

15. T. E. Wiswell and D. W. Geschke, "Risks from Circumcision during the First Month of Life Compared with Those for Uncircumcised Boys," *Pediatrics* 83 (1989): 1011–15.

16. Rosemary Romberg, personal letter of 7 January 1992.

17. Ibid.

18. T. E. Wiswell, "Circumcision—Not Prophylaxis," *Southern Medical Journal* 79 (1986): 1464.

19. Ron Nordland, Ray Wilkinson, and Ruth Marshall, "Africa in the Plague Years," *Newsweek* (24 November 1986): 44.

20. J. N. Simonsen et al., "Human Immunodeficiency Virus Infection among Men with Sexually Transmitted Diseases," *New England Journal of Medicine* 319 (4 August 1988): 277.

21. Jean L. Marx, "Circumcision May Protect against the AIDS Virus," *Science* 245 (1989): 470–71.

22. Stephen Moses, Janet E. Bradley, Nico J. D. Nagelkerke, A. R. Ronald, J. O. Ndinya-Achola, and F. A. Plummer, "Geographical Patterns of Male Circumcision Practices in Africa: Association with HIV Seroprevalence," *International Journal of Epidemiology* 19 (1990): 693–97.

23. A. J. Fink, *Circumcision: A Parent's Decision for Life* (Mountain View, Calif.: Kavanah, 1988). A single study suggests a higher incidence of non-gonococcal urethritis in circumcised men. G. L. Smith et al., "Circumcision as a Risk Factor for Urethritis in Racial Groups," *American Journal of Public Health* 77 (1987): 452–54.

24. Quoted in Marx, "Circumcision," 471.

25. Dagher, Selzer, and Lapides, "Carcinoma of the Penis," *Archives of Surgery* 85 (1962): 79–80; M. Riveros and R. Gorostiaga, "Cancer of the Penis,"

Archives of Surgery 85 (1962): 377–82; and G. J. Hardner et al., "Carcinoma of the Penis: Analysis of Therapy in 100 Consecutive Cases," *Journal of Urology* 108 (1972): 428–30.

26. American Academy of Pediatrics, *Committee on Fetus and Newborn*.

27. Edgar J. Schoen, G. Anderson, C. Bohon et al., "Report of the Task Force on Circumcision," *Pediatrics* 84 (1989): 390.

28. Edgar J. Schoen, *Pediatrics* 85 (1990): 889, bold print added.

29. Robert Dozor, "Routine Neonatal Circumcision: Boundary of Ritual and Science," *American Family Physician* 41 (1990): 822.

Chapter 9   *The Mystery of the Eighth Day*

1. Rosemary Romberg, "The Infant's and Young Child's Bill of Rights" (Anchorage: Peaceful Beginnings).

2. Joseph Katz, "The Question of Circumcision," *International Surgery* 62 (1977): 490–92.

3. These numbers are conservative, assuming approximately one million circumcised infants per year; a 1.4 percent rate of UTI if not circumcised, as in T. E. Wiswell, "Prepuce Presence," 740; and in infected infants a 2 percent death rate, much lower than the 11 percent death rate reported by J. M. Littlewood, "66 Infants with Urinary Tract Infections in First Month of Life," *Arch. Dis. Child* 47 (1972): 218.

4. C. W. McMillan, A. E. Weis, A. M. Johnson, "Acquired Coagulation Disorders in Children," *Pediatric Clinics of North America* 19 (1972): 1034.

5. L. Emmett Holt Jr. and Rustin McIntosh, *Holt Pediatrics*, 12th ed. (New York: Appleton-Century-Crofts, 1953), 125–26. An older reference is used because vitamin K administration has eliminated the problem, and so more recent research is not available.

6. To be precise, it is the bacteria in the baby's intestines that actually produce vitamin K.

7. Today we simply give babies a dose of vitamin K to prevent the problem. Also, circumcision later in life is more dangerous because it is done under general anesthesia.

8. James B. Wyngaarden and Lloyd H. Smith Jr., eds., *Cecil Textbook of Medicine* (Philadelphia: W. B. Saunders, 1982), 1003.

9. J. J. Corrigan Jr., "The Hemorrhagic Disorders," in *Practice of Pediatrics*, vol. 3, ed. V. C. Kelly (Hagerstown, Md.: Harper and Row, 1976), chap. 68, p. 7.

10. Rabbi Alfred S. Cohen, "*Brit Milah* and the Specter of AIDS," *Journal of Halacha and Contemporary Society* 17 (1989): 94.

11. H. Speert, "Circumcision of the Newborn: An Appraisal of Its Present Status," *Obstetrics and Gynecology* 2 (1953): 164–72.

12. Charles Weis, "A Worldwide Survey of the Current Practice of *Milah* (Ritual Circumcision)," *Jewish Social Studies* (January 1962), 31.

13. Today some Jewish scholars are recommending alternative procedures. See Cohen, "*Brit Milah*," 93–115.

Chapter 10   *Born Gay?*

1. Ann Lander's column, *Washington Post,* 25 April 1993, p. F6.

2. We mostly discuss male homosexuality, but the formation of female homosexuality appears to be very similar. See Gerard van den Aardweg, *Homosexuality and Hope: A Psychologist Talks about Treatment and Change* (Ann Arbor, Mich.: Servant Books, 1985).

3. Quoted by Charles Krauthammer, "Media Hype about the 'Gay Gene,'" *Washington Post,* 23 July 1993, p. A23.

4. Ibid.

5. "Het" is a reference to heterosexual, taken to be offensive.

6. Both parents are important, as documented by I. Bieber et al., *Homosexuality: A Psychoanalytic Study* (New York: Basic Books, 1962); N. L. Thomson et al., "Parent-Child Relationships and Sexual Identity in Male and Female Homosexuals and Heterosexuals," *Journal of Consulting and Clinical Psychology* 41 (1975): 120–27; W. G. Stephan, "Parental Relationships and Early Social Experiences of Activist Male Homosexuals and Male Heterosexuals," *Journal of Abnormal Psychology* 82 (1973): 506–13; M. Siegelman, "Parental Backgrounds of Male Homosexuals and Heterosexuals," *Archives of Sexual Behavior* 3 (1974): 3–18; and many others.

7. M. T. Saghir and E. Robins, *Male and Female Homosexuality: A Comprehensive Investigation* (Baltimore: Williams and Wilkins, 1973).

8. Bieber et al., *Homosexuality.*

9. There can be no doubt as to Solomon's heterosexuality. Unfortunately, however, his father's behavior with women was not as wise as his words. This may have had much to do with Solomon's later sexual insatiability and license.

10. Bieber et al., *Homosexuality.*

11. D. R. Mace, *Hebrew Marriage: A Sociological Study* (New York: Philosophical Library, 1953).

12. A. C. Kinsey et al., *Sexual Behaviour in the Human Male* (Philadelphia: W. B. Saunders, 1948), 483. See also Eliyahu Rosenheim, "Sexual Attitudes and Regulations in Judaism," in J. Money and H. Musaph, eds., *Handbook of Sexology* (Amsterdam: Excerpta Medica, 1977), 1315–23.

Chapter 11   *Sexual Musical Chairs*

1. A. P. Bell and M. S. Weinberg, *Homosexualities: A Study of Diversity among Men and Women* (New York: Simon and Schuster, 1978).

2. D. Hanson, *Homosexuality: The International Disease* (New York: L. S. Publications, 1965).

3. David P. McWhirter and Andrew M. Mattison, *The Male Couple: How Relationships Develop* (Englewood Cliffs, N.J.: Prentice-Hall, 1984).

4. Edward O. Laumann, John H. Gagnon, Robert T. Michael, and Stuart Michaels, *The Social Organization of Sexuality: Sexual Practices in the United States* (Chicago: University of Chicago Press, 1994), 217.

5. Quoted by William E. Dannemeyer, "Homosexuals in the Military," *Testimony before a Republican Research Committee Hearing* (9 December 1992), 7.

6. We owe this terminology to Bill Hybels, Senior Pastor, Willow Creek Community Church, South Barrington, Illinois.

7. van den Aardweg, *Homosexuality and Hope*, 123. He lists thirteen studies that have all found the same result.

8. Jennifer P. Schneider, "How to Recognize the Signs of Sexual Addiction," *Postgraduate Medicine* 90 (1991): 171.

9. Mart Crowley, *The Boys in the Band* (New York: Farrar, Straus, and Giroux, 1968), 178.

10. M. Quintanilla, "Teen-Agers from L.A. Schools Pack First District-Sanctioned Gay Prom," *Los Angeles Times*, 22 May 1994, p. M–1.

11. Michael and Patricia Branton, letter to editor, *Los Angeles Times* (home ed.), 29 May 1994, p. M–4.

12. Karen Mills, "Gay Pride Pioneer's Life Included Friendships, Dreams and Death," *Los Angeles Times*, 27 February 1994, part A, p. 1.

13. These people are not completely amoral (without moral values), that is, they hold that murder, theft, and dishonesty are wrong. Thus they do have moral values that they wish to impose on others but they label people who differ with their own values as "intolerant."

14. Bell and Weinberg, *Homosexualities*.

15. Lee Birk, "The Myth of Classical Homosexuality," in *Homosexual Behavior*, ed. Judd Marmor (New York: Basic Books, 1980), 266–77.

16. M. Scott Peck, *The Road Less Traveled: A New Psychology of Love, Traditional Values and Spiritual Growth* (New York: Simon & Schuster, 1978), 53.

17. van den Aardweg, *Homosexuality and Hope*, 101.

18. "Social Barriers to Prevention," in Charles F. Turner, Heather G. Miller, and Lincoln E. Moses, eds., *AIDS: Sexual Behavior and Intravenous Drug Use* (Washington, D.C.: National Academy Press, 1989), 395.

Chapter 12   AIDS—Everyone's Problem

1. "Future Shock," *Newsweek* (24 November 1986): 30–37.

2. Barbara Vobejda, "Survey Finds Most Adults Sexually Staid," *Washington Post*, 7 October 1994, p. A20.

3. At some point this graph will level off, but clearly more than 50 percent will be infected prior to their twentieth birthday.

4. E. T. Creagan, "How to Break Bad News—and Not Devastate the Patient," *Mayo Clinic Proceedings* 69 (1994): 1015–17.

5. John Donne, *Devotions upon Emergent Occasions*, no. 6., 1624.

Chapter 13   America's Sexperiment

1. *Journal of the American Medical Association* (4 April 1986).

2. Sevgi O. Aral and King K. Holmes, "Sexually Transmitted Diseases in the AIDS Era," *Scientific American* 264 (February 1991): 66.

3. *OB-GYN News* 24, 6.

4. Aral and Holmes, "Sexually Transmitted Diseases," 62–69, italics added.

5. Ibid.

6. L. Westrom, R. Joesoef, G. Reynolds et al., "Pelvic Inflammatory Disease and Fertility: A Cohort Study of 1,844 Women with Laparoscopically Verified Disease and 657 Control Women with Normal Laparoscopic Results," *Sexually Transmitted Diseases* 19 (1992): 185–92.

7. C. K. Walker, J. G. Kahn, A. E. Washington et al., "Pelvic Inflammatory Disease: Metaanalysis of Antimicrobial Regimen Efficacy," *Journal of Infectious Diseases* 168 (1993): 969–78.

8. L. Westrom, "Incidence, Prevalence, and Trends of Acute Pelvic Inflammatory Disease and Its Consequences in Industrialized Countries," *American Journal of Obstetrics and Gynecology* 138 (1980): 880–92.

9. *Note:* Chlamydia infections are treatable, but the long-term consequences of scarring of the fallopian tubes are often not reversible.

10. H. W. Wolff, *Hosea* (Philadelphia, 1974), 14–15.

Chapter 14   *A Woman's Right*

1. J. L. Carroll, K. D. Volk, and J. S. Hyde, "Differences between Males and Females in Motives for Engaging in Sexual Intercourse," *Archives of Sexual Behavior* 14 (1985): 131–39.

2. Ibid.

3. D. L. Mosher and F. D. Anderson, "Macho Personality, Sexual Aggression, and Reactions to Guided Imagery of Realistic Rape," *Journal of Research in Personality* 20 (1986): 77–94.

4. Ibid.

5. Study described in *Time* (15 August 1994): 51.

6. The *Janus Report of Sexual Behavior* (Wiley).

7. Jonathan Alter, "Beatty and Bening," *USA Weekend* (7–9 October 1994): 5.

8. C. Everett Koop, Speech to California Legislature, 6 March 1987, in Inge B. Corless and Mary Pittman-Lindeman, *AIDS: Principles, Practices, & Politics*, ref. ed. (New York: Hemisphere Publishing, 1989), 197–203.

9. Albert D. Klassen, Coin J. Williams, Eugene E. Levitt et al., "Trends in Premarital Sexual Behavior," in Charles F. Turner, Heather G. Miller, and Lincoln E. Moses, eds., *AIDS: Sexual Behavior and Intravenous Drug Use* (Washington, D.C.: National Academy Press, 1989), 553.

10. "Social Barriers to Prevention," in Turner et al., *AIDS: Sexual Behavior and Intravenous Drug Use*, 382–401.

11. *Selected Behaviors That Increase Risk for HIV Infection among High School Students—United States, 1990* 41 (Washington, D. C.: National Academy Press, 1992): 231–41.

12. Ibid.

13. Quoted by Joe S. McIlhaney Jr., *Sexuality and Sexually Transmitted Diseases* (Grand Rapids, Mich.: Baker, 1990), 59.

14. K. R. Ablow, "Sexist Remarks: Tapping the Reservoir of Male Anger," *Washington Post Health* (10 December 1991): 9, italics added.

15. *Glamour* (April 1991), 296.

16. *Cosmopolitan,* 1980.

17. V. Mary Stewart, *Sexual Freedom* (Downers Grove, Ill.: InterVarsity Press).

Chapter 15   *Our Condom Nation*

1. J. A. Catania, T. J. Coates, R. Stall, H. Turner et al., "Prevalence of AIDS-Related Risk Factors and Condom Use in the United States," *Science* 258 (1992): 1101.

2. *Medical Tribune* (8 July 1993): 12.

3. "Assessment of Street Outreach for HIV Prevention—Selected Sites, 1991–1993," *Morbidity and Mortality Weekly Report* 42 (1993): 883.

4. *USA Today,* 19 May 1992.

5. J. R. Ickovics et al., "Limited Effects of HIV Counseling and Testing for Women," *Journal of the American Medical Association* 272 (10 August 1994): 443–48.

6. D. L. Higgins et al., "Evidence for the Effects of HIV Antibody Counseling and Testing on Risk Behaviors," *Journal of the American Medical Association* 226 (1991): 2419–29.

7. N. S. Wenger et al., "Effect of HIV Antibody Testing and AIDS Education on Communication about HIV Risk and Sexual Behavior," *Annals of Internal Medicine* 117 (1992): 905–11.

8. V. I. Rickert, M. S. Hay, A. Gottlieb, and C. Bridges, "Adolescents and AIDS . . . ," *Journal of Adolescent Health Care* 10 (1989): 313.

9. Ickovics et al., "Limited Effects of HIV Counseling," 447.

10. Kathleen McCleary, "Sex, Morals and AIDS," *USA Weekend,* 27–29 December 1991, p. 5.

11. Quoted in the *National Review* (27 February 1987), 21.

12. *US News and World Report* (16 December 1991), 93.

13. U.S. Dept. of Health and Human Services, "Sexual Behavior among High School Students—United States, 1990."

14. Constance B. Wofsy, "Transmission of HIV by Prostitutes and Prevention of Spread," in P. T. Cohen, M. A. Sande, and P. A. Volberding, eds., *The AIDS Knowledge Base* (Waltham, Mass.: Medical Publishing Group, 1990), chap. 1.2.5.

15. F. D. Rolance, "Condoms: Keeping Them Safe," *Chicago Sun-Times,* 23 March 1992, p. 7.

16. S. C. Weller, "A Meta-Analysis of Condom Effectiveness in Reducing Sexually Transmitted HIV," *Social Science Medicine* 36 (1993): 1635–44; italics added.

17. As cited in "Social Barriers to Prevention," 383.

18. Public Health Service, *Healthy People 2000: National Health Promotion and Disease Prevention Objectives—Full Report, with Commentary* (Washington, D.C.: U.S. Department of Health and Human Services, Public Health Service, 1991); DHHS publication no. (PHS)91–50212.

19. *Patient Care* (15 September 1993), italics added.

20. Rufinus as cited by R. L. Fox, *Pagans and Christians* (New York: Knopf, 1989), 346.

21. Fox, *Pagans and Christians*, 345.

22. Centers for Disease Control, "Guidelines for Effective School Health Education," *Morbidity and Mortality Weekly Report* 37 (Suppl. S–2): 1–14.

Chapter 16   *Spiritual Sexuality*

1. Scholars sometimes use the term *sacrament* as a technical term to describe various formal acts of worship (communion and baptism for example) formally instituted, depending on one's tradition, by Jesus or the church. We are using the term nontechnically to describe any God-ordained act of worship, by which his grace can touch our lives.

2. M. Scott Peck, *Further Along the Road Less Traveled* (New York: Simon & Schuster, 1993), 220.

3. Adolf Guggenbuhl-Craig, *Marriage—Dead or Alive* (Zurich: Spring Publications, 1977), 43–44.

4. Ibid.

Chapter 17   *The Secret of Great Sex*

1. Aldous Huxley, *Tomorrow and Tomorrow and Tomorrow, and Other Essays* (New York: Harper and Row, 1956), 68.

2. Mark 14:36, literally, *"Abba."* Even today Jewish toddlers call their father, "Abba." See Galatians 4:6 where we, too, are called to an intimate relationship with *Abba* Father.

3. The concept of LOVE is definitely stated in the Old Testament, but it was mostly ignored by first-century Judaism.

4. C. S. Lewis, *The Four Loves* (New York: Harcourt, Brace, Jovanovich, 1960), 183.

5. Thank you, Lynn Thrush.

6. Carl Jung, *Modern Man in Search of a Soul* (New York: Harcourt, Brace and Co., 1933), 260.

7. Smiley Blanton, *Love or Perish* (New York: Simon and Schuster, 1956), 3–15.

8. Sex exercises are not inherently wrong but should always be used in the context of marriage and after issues of LOVE and a lack of LOVE are in the process of being resolved.

9. Erich Fromm, *Psychoanalysis and Religion* (New Haven: Yale University Press, 1950), 86–87.

10. Max Levin, "Sex in Modern Life," *Current Medical Digest* (September 1961): 55.

11. Ellen Ladowsky, "The Decline and Fall of Fast and Loose," *Washington Post,* 16 October 1994, p. C4.

12. Robert T. Michael, John H. Gagnon, Edward O. Laumann, and Gina Kolata, *Sex in America: A Definitive Survey* (Boston: Little, Brown, 1994), 127.

13. Edward O. Laumann, John H. Gagnon, Robert T. Michael, and Stuart Michaels, *The Social Organization of Sexuality: Sexual Practices in the United States* (Chicago: University of Chicago Press, 1994), 373.

14. Ibid., 358. Cause and effect relationships between orgasm and happiness are somewhat "chicken or the egg" issues. If a woman is anorgasmic, she is more likely to be unhappy; but also if a woman is unhappy, she is more likely to be anorgasmic.

15. Herbert J. Miles, *Sexual Happiness in Marriage* (Grand Rapids: Zondervan, 1967).

16. Sex for procreation alone has been the traditional emphasis in many churches, but the Bible definitely encourages the relational aspect of sex.

Chapter 18   *The Spirit-Mind-Body Link*

1. Cited by J. Carpi, "Relieving the Strain of Stress," *Medical World News* (May 1993): 23.

2. Sheldon Cohen, D. A. J. Tyrrell, and A. P. Smith, "Psychological Stress and Susceptibility to the Common Cold," *New England Journal of Medicine* 355 (29 August 1991): 606–12.

3. Cited in *Washington Post Health* (29 March 1994): 5.

4. J. D. Kark, S. Goldman, and L. Epstein, "Iraqi Missile Attacks on Israel: The Association of Mortality with a Life-Threatening Stressor," *Journal of the American Medical Association* 273 (19 April 1995): 1208–10.

5. H. Weiner, *Perturbing the Organism: The Biology of Stressful Experience* (Chicago: University of Chicago Press, 1992).

6. L. C. Duffy, M. A. Zielezny, J. R. Marshall et al., "Relevance of Major Stress Events as an Indicator of Disease Activity Prevalence in Inflammatory Bowel Disease," *Behavioral Medicine* 17 (1991): 101–10.

7. J. H. Markovitz, K. A. Matthews, W. B. Kannel et al., "Psychological Predictors of Hypertension in the Framingham Study: Is There Tension in Hypertension?" *Journal of the American Medical Association* 270 (1993): 2439–43.

8. J. J. Lynch et al., "Psychological Aspects of Cardiac Arrhythmia," *American Heart Journal* 93 (1977): 645.

9. J. H. Medalie et al., "Angina Pectoris among 10,000 Men: 5 Year Incidence and Univariate Analysis," *American Journal of Medicine* 55 (1973): 583.

10. K. A. Matthews, "Coronary Heart Disease and Type A. Behaviors: Update on and Alternative to the Booth-Kewley and Friedman (1987) Quantitative Review," *Psycho Bulletin* 104 (1988): 373–80; S. C. Jacobs, R. Friedman, M. Mittleman et al., "9-Fold Increased Risk of Myocardial Infarction

Following Psychological Stress as Assessed by a Case-Control Study," *Circulation* 86, suppl. (1992): 1–198.

11. R. Adler, K. MacRitchie, and G. L. Engle, "Psychologic Process and Ischemic Stroke (Occlusive Cerebrovascular Disease): Observations on 32 Men with 35 Strokes," *Psychosomatic Medicine* 33 (1971): 1.

12. R. L. Gallon, ed., *The Psychosomatic Approach to Illness* (New York: Elsevier Biomedical, 1982), 168–72.

13. Ibid.

14. Ibid.

15. B. Winsa, H. O. Adami, R. Bergstrom et al. "Stressful Life Events and Grave's Disease," *Lancet* 338 (1991): 1475–79.

16. R. S. Surwit, S. L. Ross, and M. N. Feingloss, "Stress, Behavior, and Glucose Control in Diabetes Mellitus," in *Stress, Coping, and Disease*, eds. P. McCabe et al. (Hillsdale, N.J., 1991), 97–117; and B. Hagglof, I. Blom, G. Dahlquist et al., "The Swedish Childhood Diabetes Study: Indications of Severe Psychological Stress as a Risk Factor for Type I (Insulin-Dependent) Diabetes Mellitus in Childhood," *Diabetologia* 34 (1991): 579–83.

17. Y. Nakai et al., "Alexithymic Features of the Patients with Chronic Pancreatitis," *Proceedings of the Fourth Congress of the International College of Psychosomatic Medicine* (Basel: Karger, 1977).

18. A. Wilson, I. Hickie, A. Llowyd et al., "Longitudinal Study of Outcome of Chronic Fatigue Syndrome," *British Journal of Medicine* 308 (1994): 756. *Note:* This disease is controversial and hard to classify, but psychological factors appear to be the main predictors of outcome in this illness.

19. S. A. Isenberg, P. M. Lehrer, and S. Hochron, "The Effects of Suggestions and Emotional Arousal on Pulmonary Function in Asthma: A Review and a Hypothesis Regarding Vagal Mediation," *Psychosomatic Medicine* 54 (1992): 192–216.

20. R. Glaser, J. K. Kiecolt-Glaser, E. H. Bonneau et al., "Stress-Induced Modulation of the Immune Response to Recombinant Hepatitis B Vaccine," *Psychosomatic Medicine* 54 (1992): 22–29.

21. H. Weiner, "Social and Psychobiological Factors in Autoimmune Disease," in *Psychoneuroimmunology*, ed. R. Adler, O. L. Felten, and N. Cohen (Orlando, Fla.: Academic Press, 1991), 995–1011; and G. F. Solomon, "Emotional and Personality Factors in the Onset and Course of Autoimmune Disease, Particularly Rheumatoid Arthritis," in *Psychoneuroimmunology*, ed. R. Adler (New York: Academic Press, 1981), 174–75.

22. M. S. Juhn, "Myasthenia Gravis," *Postgraduate Medicine* 94 (October 1993): 162.

23. Sheldon Cohen, D. A. J. Tyrrell, and A. P. Smith, *New England Journal of Medicine* 355 (29 August 1991): 606–12.

24. J. Kiecolt-Glaser and R. Glaser, "Stress and Immune Function in Humans," in *Psychoneuroimmunology*, ed. R. Adler, O. L. Felten, and N. Cohen, 849–67.

25. T. H. Holmes, "Psychosocial and Psychophysiological Studies of Tuberculosis," in *Physiological Correlates of Psychological Disorders*, ed. R. R. Greenfield (Madison, Wisc.: University of Wisconsin, 1962), 239–55.

26. R. J. Meyer and R. J. Haggerty, "Streptococcal Infections in Families: Factors Altering Individual Susceptibility," *Pediatrics* 29 (1962): 539.

27. A. M. Jacobson, T. C. Manschrech, and E. Silverberg, "Behavioral Treatment for Raynaud's Disease: A Comparative Study with Long-Term Follow-Up," *American Journal of Psychiatry* 136 (1979): 844.

28. R. L. Horne and R. S. Picard, "Psychosocial Risk Factors for Lung Cancer," *Psychosomatic Medicine* 41 (1979): 503.

29. S. Lehrer, "Life Change and Gastric Cancer," *Psychosomatic Medicine* 42 (1980): 499.

30. T. J. Jacobs and E. Charles, "Life Events and the Occurrence of Cancer in Children," *Psychosomatic Medicine* 42 (1980): 11.

31. D. Spiegel, H. Kraemer, J. Bloom, and E. Gottheil, "Effect of Psychosocial Treatment on Survival of Patients with Metastatic Breast Cancer," *Lancet* 339 (1991): 888–91.

32. R. B. Shekelle et al., "Psychological Depression and 17-Year Risk of Death from Cancer," *Psychosomatic Medicine* 43 (1981): 117.

Chapter 19   *Public Enemy Number One*

1. www.cdc.gov/od/oc/media/fact/cardiova.htm

2. T. Gordon and W. B. Kannel, "Obesity and Cardiovascular Disease: The Framingham Heart Study," *Clinics in Endocrinology and Metabolism* 5 (1976): 367.

3. W. B. Kannel and T. Gordon, "Physiological and Medical Concomitants of Obesity: The Framingham Heart Study," in *Obesity in America* (Washington, D.C.: Government Printing Office, 1979), 125.

4. P. L. Schnall, J. E. Schwartz, P. A. Landsbergis et al., "A Longitudinal Study of Job Strain and Ambulatory Blood Pressure: Results from a Three-Year Follow-Up," *Psychosomatic Medicine* 60 (1998): 697. Actual average elevation of 11/7 mm Hg (high stress) and drop of 5/3 mm Hg (switch to low stress).

5. M. F. Muldoon, T. B. Herbert, S. M. Patterson et al., "Effects of Acute Psychological Stress on Serum Lipid Levels, Hemoconcentration, and Blood Viscosity," *Archives of Internal Medicine* 155 (1995): 615.

6. P. P. Vitaliano, J. M. Scanlan, C. Krenz et al., "Psychological Distress, Caregiving, and Metabolic Variables," *J Gerontol B Psychol Sci Soc Sci* 51 (1996): 290.

7. Muldoon et al., "Effects of Acute Psychological Stress," 615.

8. J. H. Markovitz, K. A. Matthews, J. Kiss et al., "Effects of Hostility on Platelet Reactivity to Psychological Stress in Coronary Heart Disease Patients and in Healthy Controls," *Psychosomatic Medicine* 58 (1996): 143.

9. W. J. Kop, K. Hamulyak, C. Pernot, and A. Appels, "Relationship of Blood Coagulation and Fibrinolysis to Vital Exhaustion," *Psychosomatic Medicine* 60 (1998): 352.

10. Based on data from R. H. Rahe and M. Romo, "Recent Life Changes and the Onset of Myocardial Infarction and Coronary Death in Helsinki," in *Life, Stress and Illness,* ed. E. K. E. Gunderson and R. H. Rahe (Springfield, Ill.: Charles C. Thomas, 1974), 111; and T. Theorell and R. H. Rahe, "Psychosocial Characteristics of Subjects with Myocardial Infarction in Stockholm," in *Life, Stress and Illness,* 96.

Chapter 20   *The Stress-Free Life*

1. This has been reported to be a favorite saying of Hans Selye, father of stress theory.

2. Gallup poll of 1,011 adults in Barbara Paulsen, "A Nation Out of Balance," *Hippocrates* (October 1994): 29–32.

3. Quoted in Paulsen, "A Nation Out of Balance," 30.

4. R. Svendsrod, "Locus of Control and Life at Work," in H. Ursin and R. Murison, eds., *Biological and Psychological Basis of Psychosomatic Disease* (Oxford, England: Pergamon Press, 1983), 137.

5. J. Rodin, "Managing the Stress of Aging: The Role of Control and Coping," in S. Levine and H. Ursin, eds., *Coping and Health* (New York: Plenum Press, 1980).

6. H. M. Lefcourt, "The Function of the Illusions of Control and Freedom," *American Psychologist* 28 (1973): 424–25.

7. K. I. Maton, "The Stress-Buffering Role of Spiritual Support: Cross-Sectional and Prospective Investigation," *Journal for the Scientific Study of Religion* 28 (1989): 310–23.

8. H. G. Koenig, J. N. Kvale, and C. Ferrel, "Religion and Well-Being in Later Life," *The Gerontologist* 28 (1988): 18–28.

9. J. J. Lindenthal, J. K. Myers, M. P. Pepper, and M. S. Stern, "Mental Status and Religious Behavior," *Journal for the Scientific Study of Religion* 9 (1970): 143–49; see also R. Stark, "Psychopathology and Religious Commitment," *Review of Religious Research* 12 (1971): 165–76.

10. R. W. Williams, D. B. Larson, R. E. Buckler, R. C. Heckmann, and C. M. Pyle, "Religion and Psychological Distress in a Community Sample," *Social Science Medicine* 32 (1991): 1257–62.

11. H. G. Theiel, D. Parker, and T. A. Bruce, "Stress Factors and the Risk of Myocardial Infarction," *Journal of Psychosomatic Research* 17 (1973): 43–57.

12. Richard J. Foster, *Celebration of Discipline: Paths to Spiritual Growth* (New York: Harper and Row, 1978), 84.

Chapter 21   *The Faith Factor*

1. Susan Parker, "Experts Call Spirituality an Untapped Therapy," *Internal Medicine News* (15 January 1996), 34.

2. G. W. Comstock and K. B. Partridge, "Church Attendance and Health," *Journal of Chronic Disease* 25 (1972): 665–72. *Note:* These reductions remained even after controlling for the effects of smoking.

3. T. E. Oxman, D. H. Freeman Jr., and E. D. Manheimer, "Lack of Social Participation or Religious Strength and Comfort as Risk Factors for Death after Cardiac Surgery in the Elderly," *Psychosomatic Medicine* 57 (1995): 5–15.

4. P. Pressman, J. S. Lyons, D. S. Larson, and J. J. Strain, "Religious Belief, Depression, and Ambulation Status in Elderly Women with Broken Hips," *American Journal of Psychiatry* 147 (1990): 758–60.

5. D. M. Zuckerman, S. V. Kasl, and A. M. Ostfeld, "Psychosocial Predictors of Mortality among the Elderly Poor," *American Journal of Epidemiology* 119 (1984): 410–23.

6. Note that both phrases are identical in the original Greek.

7. Alzina Stone Dale, *The Outline of Sanity* (Grand Rapids, Mich.: Eerdmans, 1982), 149.

8. Kim Sue Lia Perkes, *U.S. News and World Report* (4 April 1994), 54.

9. Redford and Virginia Williams, *Anger Kills* (New York: Harper Collins, 1993), 184.

10. J. S. Levin, "Religion and Health: Is There an Association, Is It Valid, and Is It Causal?" *Social Science Medicine* 38 (1994): 1476.

11. Williams, *Anger Kills*, 181.

12. Cited by David B. Larson and Susan S. Larson, *The Forgotten Factor in Physical and Mental Health: What Does the Research Show?* (Available through the Christian Medical & Dental Society, P.O. Box 830689, Richardson, TX 75083–0689). This publication and an annotated bibliography, also available through the CMDS, are excellent, scholarly, in-depth reviews of this subject.

Chapter 22   *Danger—Anger*

1. See Carol Tavris, *Anger: The Misunderstood Emotion* (New York: Simon and Schuster, 1989) for a review of this research. We are much indebted to her summary of the subject.

2. Ebbe Ebbesen, Birt Duncan, and Vladimir Konecni, "Effects of Content of Verbal Aggression on Future Verbal Aggression: A Field Experiment," *Journal of Experimental Social Psychology* 11 (1975): 192–204.

Chapter 23   *The High Cost of Getting Even*

1. Williams, *Anger Kills*, 186.

2. Aristotle, *Nicomachean Ethics* 1126a, 2.

Chapter 24 *Mind over Madder*

1. Neil Clark Warren, *Make Anger Your Ally* (Colorado Springs: Focus on the Family Publishing, 1990), 153.

2. Seymour Feshbach, "The Catharsis Hypothesis and Some Consequences of Interaction with Aggression and Neutral Play Objects," *Journal of Personality* 24 (1959): 449–62.

Chapter 25 *Tears*

1. S. Fishman, "Relationships among and Older Adult's Life Review, Ego Integrity, and Death Anxiety," *Int. Psychogeriatr.* 4, suppl. 2 (1992): 267–77.

2. J. A. Thorson and F. C. Powell, "Meanings of Death and Intrinsic Religiosity," *Journal of Clinical Psychology* 46 (1990): 379–91.

3. D. N. McIntosh, R. C. Silver, C. B. Wortman, "Religion's Role in Adjustment to a Negative Life Event: Coping with the Loss of a Child," *J. Pers. Soc. Psychol.* 65 (1993): 812–21.

4. Raymond Brown, *The Gospel According to John* (New York: Doubleday, 1966), 423.

5. Leon Morris, *The Gospel According to John* (Grand Rapids, Mich.: Eerdmans, 1971), 542.

6. Quoted in Sheldon Vanauken, *A Severe Mercy* (New York: Bantam Books, 1977), 189.

7. Henry Maudsley, quoted by I. Gregory and D. J. Smeltzer, *Psychiatry: Essentials of Clinical Practice* (Boston: Little, Brown, 1983), 321.

8. This is an edited version. It is a sad reality of American life, and this analogy is not intended to imply that this is a good change.

Chapter 26 *Don't Shoot for the Moon*

1. This is a sad reality of American life, and this analogy is not intended to imply that this is a good change.

Chapter 27 *Are You Wearing a Parachute?*

1. We owe this illustration to Ray Comfort, *Hell's Best Kept Secret* (Pittsburgh: Whitaker House, 1989), 10–11.

Chapter 28 *The Soul Set Free*

1. Carl Jung, *Modern Man in Search of a Soul* (New York: Harcourt, Brace, and Co., 1933), 273.

2. Ibid., 260–62.